Using Qualitative Research

For Churchill Livingstone:

Commissioning Editor: Mary Law
Project Manager: Gail Murray
Project Development Manager: Dinah Thom

Using Qualitative Research

A Practical Introduction for Occupational and Physical Therapists

Edited by

Karen Whalley Hammell MSc PhD DipCOT
Freelance writer, Saskatchewan, Canada

Christine Carpenter BA MA DipPT
Doctoral Candidate and Senior Instructor, School of Rehabilitation Sciences, University of British Columbia, Vancouver, Canada

Isabel Dyck BA MA PhD DipCOT
Associate Professor, School of Rehabilitation Sciences, University of British Columbia, Vancouver, Canada

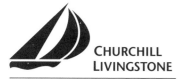

CHURCHILL
LIVINGSTONE

EDINBURGH LONDON NEW YORK PHILADELPHIA ST LOUIS SYDNEY TORONTO 2000

CHURCHILL LIVINGSTONE
An imprint of Harcourt Publishers Limited

© Harcourt Publishers Limited 2000

⤍ is a registered trademark of Harcourt Publishers Limited

First published 2000

ISBN 0 443 06232 3

British Library of Cataloguing in Publication Data
A catalogue record for this book is available from the British Library.

Library of Congress Cataloging in Publication Data
A catalog record for this book is available from the Library of Congress.

Note
Medical knowledge is constantly changing. As new information becomes available, changes in treatment, procedures, equipment and the use of drugs become necessary. The editors and the publishers have, as far as it is possible, taken care to ensure that the information given in this text is accurate and up to date. However, readers are strongly advised to confirm that the information complies with the latest legislation and standards of practice.

The publisher's policy is to use **paper manufactured from sustainable forests**

Printed in China

Contents

Contributors

Christine Carpenter BA MA DipPT

Doctoral Candidate and Senior Instructor, School of Rehabilitation Sciences, University of British Columbia, Vancouver, Canada

Chris was educated as a physiotherapist in Liverpool, England, and received her other degrees at the University of British Columbia, Vancouver, Canada. She worked clinically in rehabilitation, with a specific interest in spinal cord injury, before becoming a senior instructor at the School of Rehabilitation Sciences, Division of Physical Therapy. Currently completing her PhD in Educational Studies, Chris's interests are in provision of care issues in rehabilitation settings, client-centred practice, health-care ethics, clinical education and teaching instructional skills.

Isabel Dyck BA MA PhD DipCOT

Associate Professor, School of Rehabilitation Sciences, University of British Columbia, Vancouver, Canada

Isabel's occupational therapy education was completed in Oxford, England, after which she practised in England, Canada and India. Her BA and MA are in Social Anthropology from the University of Manchester, England, and her PhD is in Social Geography from Simon Fraser University, Canada. She has published extensively on methodological issues in research, particularly from a feminist perspective, and her research concerns women with disabilities and immigrant settlement issues, including family reconstitution and health care.

Sue Forwell BSc(OT) MA

Senior Instructor, School of Rehabilitation Sciences, University of British Columbia, Vancouver, Canada

Sue received her bachelor's degree in Occupational Therapy in 1982 from the University of Western Ontario, Canada, and her master's degree from the University of Southern California, USA, in 1989. She has worked extensively with adults with neurological impairments. Currently, Sue holds a position as Senior Instructor and Fieldwork Coordinator in the Division of Occupational Therapy, the University of British Columbia, is Chair of the University Fieldwork Coordinators of Canada, and is Coordinator of the Education Division for the Canadian Association of Occupational Therapists.

Karen Whalley Hammell MSc PhD DipCOT

Freelance writer, Saskatchewan, Canada

Karen was educated as an occupational therapist in Liverpool, later gaining her Master of Science degree in Rehabilitation Studies (with Distinction), from the University of Southampton, England, and a Doctor of Philosophy degree in Interdisciplinary Studies (Rehabilitation Sciences, Anthropology and Sociology) from the University of British Columbia, Canada. Currently writing in Saskatchewan, Karen's special interests are in spinal cord injuries, disability theory, client-centred practice and occupation theory. She is the author of the 1995 book *Spinal Cord Injury Rehabilitation*.

Lyn Jongbloed BSc(OT) PhD (Canada) MA Dip(OT) (South Africa)

Associate Professor, School of Rehabilitation Sciences, University of British Columbia, Vancouver, Canada
From a background of clinical experience among people with spinal cord injuries, strokes and chronic mental illnesses, Lyn's current research focuses on the interrelationships between disability and the social, economic and political environments. She has recently co-authored a book entitled *Disability and Social Policy in Canada*.

Sue Stanton BSR(OT) MA Dip(OT)

Senior Instructor, School of Rehabilitation Sciences, University of British Columbia, Vancouver, Canada
Sue is an occupational therapy graduate from New Zealand who is a faculty member of the School of Rehabilitation Sciences at the University of British Columbia. A co-author of three chapters in two occupational therapy texts, she has published articles relating to stroke, organizational change and occupational therapy fieldwork. Sue was a consultant in the development of two new occupational therapy programmes in New Zealand in 1990, and regularly coaches faculty in developing instructional skills.

Melinda Suto BS(OT) MA

Senior Instructor, School of Rehabilitation Sciences, University of British Columbia, Vancouver, Canada
Melinda received a bachelor's degree in occupational therapy at San Jose State University, California, and earned her Master of Arts degree in the Department of Occupational Therapy at the University of Southern California under the supervision of Dr Gelya Frank. Melinda is completing her PhD in Educational Studies at the University of British Columbia. Her interests include community mental health issues, and concepts of leisure and time use, with particular focus on immigrants within Canada.

Toby Wendland BSc (Kinesiology), BScOT

Practising occupational therapist, USA
Toby undertook his occupational therapy education at the University of British Columbia, Canada. After gaining experience in a diversity of clinical and geographical settings in the USA (including arthritis and geriatric care, neurological and orthopaedic rehabilitation, and paediatrics), he is currently employed as a school-based paediatric OT. His special interests are in neurological rehabilitation and paediatric therapy.

Preface

There is a growing enthusiasm for qualitative research in the health sciences. This reflects the recognition that traditional quantitative research approaches have rendered client and consumer voices invisible and that they are unable to illuminate the experience of (and thus the appropriate response to) illness, injury or disability. Qualitative methods are seen by many health-care professionals as a means to explore the complexities of issues arising from clinical practice, or of living with a disability.

In 1995 and 1996 we formed a discussion group at the School of Rehabilitation Sciences at the University of British Columbia, Vancouver, Canada, for faculty members and graduate students who had an interest in qualitative research. Our discussions centred on existing published papers and texts, but it quickly became apparent that no single text was available to address issues that was both informative about qualitative research and relevant to a rehabilitation context. Indeed, it became apparent to us that those rehabilitation researchers who use a qualitative methodology draw from a diversity of sources from within such disciplines as education, women's studies, nursing, anthropology and sociology. *Using Qualitative Research: A Practical Introduction for Occupational and Physical Therapists* represents our joint effort to create a text which will fill the current gap in the literature.

This book aims, therefore, to provide a practical introduction to qualitative research for undergraduate and postgraduate students, researchers and clinicians in both physical and occupational therapy, as well as for others involved in either rehabilitation or disability studies. It will be useful both to those involved in research and to those who seek a clearer understanding of qualitative research reports now appearing in the leading therapy and disability journals.

In an effort to create a text that is firmly grounded within current rehabilitation philosophy and concerns, the book assumes a problem-based approach. Each contributing author discusses a specific research project, and together these form the basis for an understanding of the most important issues in qualitative research. It is our hope and intention that this will provide an introduction to using qualitative research that is both practical and useful, highlighting issues of ethics, methods and analysis through examination of our own research experiences.

Karen Whalley Hammell
Christine Carpenter
Vancouver 1999   Isabel Dyck

1

Introduction to qualitative research in occupational therapy and physical therapy

Karen Hammell   Chris Carpenter

KEY POINTS

qualitative research methodology in occupational therapy and physical therapy – characteristics and underlying assumptions; 'fit' of methodology to research questions; congruency with contemporary professional philosophies; contributions to theory development

OVERVIEW

In this chapter we provide an introductory overview of qualitative research, grounded on the premise that qualitative research addresses a different type of question than is possible using more traditional, quantitative methods. The focus of the chapter will be to explore why we might choose to conduct qualitative research in occupational therapy and physical therapy, and to establish the congruency of qualitative research methodologies with current interest within both our professions in client-centred, community-based (contextual) practice and contemporary health-care ethics. Central themes will be the contribution qualitative research can make to the development of strong theoretical frameworks for professional practice, and the related need to inform practice through an improved understanding of the perspective of the individuals who experience chronic illness or disability.

TERMINOLOGY AND CLASSIFICATIONS

The use of the terms 'methods' and 'methodology' is not consistent across academic disciplines. In this book the term 'methodology' will be used to refer to the philosophical, conceptual and theoretical aspects that underpin the approaches employed to develop knowledge. The research 'methods' are defined as being the actual techniques and strategies employed to acquire knowledge and manipulate data (Cancian 1992).

Many variations on the basic approach to qualitative inquiry have evolved over the 100-year history of qualitative research (Peters 1996). Perhaps responding to prevailing reductionistic traditions, many researchers using a qualitative methodology have found it difficult to resist the temptation to demarcate individual research techniques, and thereafter to prescribe rigid criteria for adherents to follow. In reading existing qualitative texts, it is common to encounter subdivisions, including (but not limited to) ethnography, ethnology, ethnoscience, phenomenology, life history, symbolic interactionism, case studies, grounded theory, discourse analysis and narrative approaches. Although some researchers view these philosophies and theories as separate qualitative research approaches, few writers are able to agree on precise definitions or applications, or to differentiate between whether they understand these to be research methods or methodologies.

Suspicious of attempts to submerge fairly straightforward and accessible research approaches within complex and élitist language and theories, in this book we take the view that these various approaches are tools, not doctrines, and that, as researchers, we should

use the most appropriate tools available, responding to the context and content of the research data as they emerge. This position is defended by the desire to engage in a research process characterized by 'flexibility and freedom within guidelines' (Hasselkus 1991, p. 7). Accordingly, we take the position that 'qualitative research' is an umbrella term used to refer to a number of theoretical perspectives that share certain assumptions or characteristics (Carpenter 1997). These assumptions are outlined below.

THE LEGACY OF WESTERN PHILOSOPHY

The early Greek philosopher Plato established a charter for a dualistic world view that became ingrained in Western philosophy; for example, reason and emotion; permanence and change; heaven and earth; mind and body. Reflecting this world view, for succeeding centuries the search for knowledge of natural phenomena has been dominated by the dualism – or dichotomy – later expounded by Descartes, that posits the mind and body as being distinct and separate, and claiming that an objective world (or reality) exists outside subjective human perceptions (Holman 1993). From this dualistic perspective the search for 'objectivity' became prized, and reductionist research strategies were developed to minimize complexity among variables, to enable replicability by other researchers, and to reduce observations to numerical form; thus these approaches to research are generally known as 'quantitative'. For example, a therapist might wish to evaluate whether a prescribed exercise regimen for clients with a total hip replacement reduces the number of days for which a walking frame ('walker') must be used. Such a study would require the therapist/researcher to control such independent variables as the ages and genders of the research subjects, so that the dependent variable (the number of days for which a walker was used) could be identified and measured without other varying influences to confuse the findings. Thus, quantitative methods are at their most effective when the subject under study may be so controlled as to eliminate the possibility of other influences upon the research findings; the research subjects themselves are, ideally, homogeneous and passive (Holman 1993).

THE LIMITATIONS OF REDUCTIONISM

There can be little doubt that the use of reductionist strategies has contributed an enormous wealth of knowledge to modern biomedicine, and thereafter to the professions of occupational therapy and physical therapy. However, within both our disciplines, as well as within the professions of nursing and medicine, the limitations of quantitative methodologies to address the questions that are pertinent to our clients and contemporary clinical practice are being recognized and contested.

Holman (1993) notes that chronic illnesses are 'the most prevalent contemporary medical problems' (p. 31) for which conventional bio-medical research has contributed little useful insight – an observation that would un-doubtedly be supported by many occupational therapy and physical therapy clinicians. Holman argues that the repertoire of investigatory techniques must be expanded if the degree of knowledge which is essential to the manage-ment of disability and chronicillness – by both clients and their health-care professionals – is to be attained.

Further, within occupational therapy and physical therapy research, controlled experi-ments that reduce occupation or movement to a simple cause-and-effect relationship lose sight of the person and the reasons underlying either engagement in occupation or movement. Experimental approaches are based on the assumption that people with the same injury, disease or degree of disability will have the same rehabilitation outcome: a fallacy few experienced clinicians would support. For example, how the hand is used following a tendon repair will depend upon more than physiology: sociocultural and economic factors, family roles and expectations, personal priorities and values, the meaning of the injury to the

client and even the weather may influence how the hand will be used. This complex equation of personal meanings and contextual contingencies relates to the uniqueness and holism of our professions, and speaks to the need for research tools that go beyond the reductionism appropriate to the physical sciences.

The meanings constructed by the use of the terms 'health', 'disease' and 'disability' are generally understood to be the consequences of the interaction of multiple forces, including (but not limited to) biology, the physical environment, social and economic circumstances and psychological state (Holman 1993). The relative influence of these various factors will change over time, as will their combined effects. To achieve an understanding of health, disease and disability that goes beyond the purely rudimentary, we need to employ research methods that capture degrees of complexity beyond the scope of quantitative research.

Including qualitative approaches

Qualitative research provides a more holistic approach to problems pertinent to the rehabilitation disciplines. A study conducted by Keysor, Sparling and Riegger-Krugh (1998) highlights this difference between the two traditions. Their research was conducted with young and middle-aged adults who had sustained severe injuries during athletics and who, as a result of the early onset of osteoarthritis in the affected joints, had to change and modify their activities and lifestyles. The researchers recognized that the processes of learning and problem solving necessary to integrate the disability resulting from osteoarthritis into individual clients' daily lives had not been addressed by the majority of current research studies. Their literature review clearly showed that quantitative research has contributed significantly to the understanding of the prevalence and risk factors of osteoarthritis, the mechanisms of pathology, psychological and sociological predictors of pain and disability, and self-care management, but little was known about the individual's experience of living with this pathology. Furthermore, most osteoarthritis research, whether quantitative or qualitative, addressed issues experienced by older adults (over 55 years). This qualitative study, which involved four participants, revealed their struggle to adapt to the multifactorial nature of their condition, when this could not be attributed to a general ageing process. Their struggle involved pain, loss of function, fear, social isolation, and feelings of helplessness, loss of self-identity and of perceived control. The authors contend that qualitative studies such as this enable rehabilitation therapists to understand some of the complexities involved in living with osteoarthritis at an earlier age. This understanding enhances their ability effectively to assist this unique group of clients to learn the interventions and strategies they need to optimize their function, quality of life and health in the context of their own lives and experiences.

THE COMPLEMENTARITY OF QUALITATIVE AND QUANTITATIVE METHODOLOGIES

Writing in the *Journal of Clinical Epidemiology*, Holman (1993) argues that 'true understanding in medicine cannot be achieved without adding qualitative methods to the research arsenal' (p. 35). However, although theorists advocate that physical therapists should become familiar with the tenets of both quantitative and qualitative approaches in order to increase their options in conducting research relevant to clinical practice (Shepard et al 1993), Holman observes that within the medical professions 'the almost sole recognition given to quantitative methods has trained students inadequately, established flawed standards of practice and research, and delayed the development of essential medical knowledge' (p. 35). It could be argued that the therapy professions have perpetuated a similarly narrow perspective of research possibilities.

Although qualitative and quantitative approaches may be complementary – as will be demonstrated in Chapter 2 – it has been noted that, rather than developing skills and expertise in both fields and thereafter utilizing the

approach best suited to their problem, researchers in the past have spent inordinate amounts of time and energy justifying their preference for one or other approach, and pointing out the deficiencies of the other (see, for example, Field & Morse 1985). The idea that one approach is inherently and in all circumstances superior to another leads to a narrow-minded allegiance to one way of thinking: the antithesis of the open-minded qualities demanded of good researchers. In Chapter 2, Lyn Jongbloed demonstrates how the characteristics of qualitative research informed a study of women with multiple sclerosis through the generation of rich data about the individual, both in context and in interaction with the environment (social, political, economic and physical), and how this understanding shaped the questions (and categories of possible answers) for the quantitative component of the study.

Creswell (1998) observes that 'Qualitative inquiry represents a legitimate mode of social and human science exploration without apology or comparisons to quantitative research. Good models of qualitative inquiry demonstrate the rigour, difficulty, and time-consuming nature of this approach' (p. 9). It is our intention in this book to demonstrate the applicability of qualitative methods to certain sorts of questions and research contexts, without claiming the superiority of one approach or another for addressing all research questions within our academic and professional disciplines. In Chapter 10 we will discuss the development of evaluative criteria specific to qualitative research.

INTRODUCING QUALITATIVE RESEARCH

Qualitative research asks different kinds of questions from those posed within reductionist traditions, seeks systematically to describe and interpret issues and phenomena, and to generate new concepts and theories (Carpenter 1997). The researcher does not seek to test preordained hypotheses or relationships between data but rather, examines the data for patterns, common themes and relationships between phenomena, returning to the data to test these emerging theories, so that research is an ongoing, cyclical process until understanding is achieved (Bogdan & Biklen 1998). This cyclical interrelationship between theory and data will be explored further by Isabel Dyck in Chapter 8.

Creswell (1998, p. 17) notes that, whereas quantitative questions 'ask "why" and look for comparisons of groups, or a relationship between variables, with the intent of establishing an association, relationship, or cause and effect', in a qualitative study the research often starts with the question 'how' or 'what', 'so that the initial forays into the topic describe what is going on' (p. 17). The use of qualitative research methods to ask different types of questions within rehabilitation practice is central to Chris Carpenter's research, discussed in Chapter 3.

The history of qualitative research

It is proposed that statistical logic and an experimental approach cannot be considered appropriate for studying the meanings and motives that underlie everyday life (Barnes 1992). Qualitative research methods arose from the tradition within anthropology of understanding, describing, interpreting, translating and presenting the inside, or 'native point of view' (Marcus & Fischer 1986, p. 25). 'Qualitative research offers a valuable and time-tested approach to the study of subjective experience' (Peters 1996, p. 146).

Anthropologists traditionally spend long periods of time living with the subjects of their studies to try to gain a deep understanding of their social organization and way of viewing the world. However, constrained by time and money, qualitative researchers in many disciplines (notably education, sociology,

'Qualitative traditions have grown out of a long-standing concern about how to best study and represent human life and human action as meaningful activity. These approaches aim to describe the complexity of human experience in its context and emphasize describing daily events of peoples' lives in their own words' (Spencer et al 1993, p. 304).

nursing and women's studies) commonly use open-ended interviewing and observation of everyday activities as their primary data-gathering tools.

Methods

Qualitative research is pluralistic, comprising a variety of approaches that reflect both philosophical and epistemological positions and the demands of the specific research context. In Chapter 4, for example, Melinda Suto describes her use of various data collection strategies, including participant observation, in her study of people with schizophrenia. Participant observation simply means that the observer participates in the daily life of the people under study. Several of the contributors to this book made use of the ethnographic interview: an in-depth, semi-structured and interactive interview with lines of questioning designed to probe specific areas of interest. These interviews are informed by the researchers' previous experience and knowledge of the issue being studied, and by their theoretical perspectives and interests, and are shaped situationally by reflecting upon what is being said by the participants. In Chapter 5, Sue Stanton demonstrates the use of in-depth interviews to gain insight into the perspectives of couples, demonstrating how these insights can be used to inform the delivery of client-centred services. Further, in Chapter 9, Toby Wendland and Karen Hammell demonstrate how an exercise in qualitative methods – conducting an ethnographic interview – may be used as a tool for undergraduate students to understand another person's life.

Philosophy

Fundamental to qualitative methodology is a concern to describe and understand how people make sense of their lives through an exploration of their perspectives and everyday realities. This gives credence to people's beliefs, value systems and the meanings with which they make sense of their lives and experiences. Further, each study participant is viewed as if with a wide-angled lens, enabling a deeper understanding of the interrelationships between them and their complex social and physical environments. Rather than seeking to exclude environmental contingencies, qualitative researchers believe that people are inseparable from their contexts or environments, whether these are social, cultural, physical, economic, political, legal or historical.

Qualitative methods thus provide the researcher with tools to examine social settings and to gain an understanding of the meanings attributed to events by human beings.

Recognizing the cooperative and interactive nature of qualitative inquiry, the term 'subject' – usually employed in quantitative research to denote those who are the objects of inquiry – is dropped in favour of terms such as 'participant' or 'co-researcher'. This attempts to reflect the active role of those researched in any research endeavour, and to remind the researcher of the respect due to those who consent to share information about their lives. Thus a philosophical and conceptual shift transforms the object of study into a participant (Peters 1996): a stance which positively reflects the ethics underpinning our professions.

SELECTING A METHODOLOGY

Fundamentally, however, the choice of a research methodology should be informed by the nature of the problem it seeks to address. If we are asking such questions as 'How many?' 'How far?' 'How big?', then careful, numerical measurements, statistical analysis and reductionistic approaches are clearly the most appropriate. However, if instead we wish to know such things as 'What is it like to be paralysed?' 'What motivates participation in certain activities?' 'What contributes to perceptions of quality in living?' – questions that pertain to values, beliefs, motivations, person–environment interactions, human behaviour and meanings – then quantitative methodologies are clearly inadequate and qualitative methodologies must be used to explore these issues from the perspectives of the study participants them-selves. Qualitative methods provide a 'different way of answering different questions' (Shepard et al 1993, p. 95).

When are qualitative methods appropriate?

Qualitative methods are appropriate when the research question pertains to understanding or describing a phenomenon about which little is known; when seeking to understand the 'inside' point of view of the study participants; and when context is integral to the question (Bogdan & Biklen 1998). A qualitative methodology is also appropriate when there is only a small number of potential study participants (Krefting 1989). For example, the small number of survivors with the highest levels of spinal cord injury meant that the potential sample group for Karen Hammell's study in the Vancouver area was a small one (see Chapter 6).

The actual number of people included in a study will depend upon such factors as the purpose of the research and the methods being used. Many researchers cease to recruit new participants at the point at which the data become 'saturated', that is, when no new themes are emerging: when new stories confirm what is already understood while adding only slight individual variations; and when the researcher has exploited the opportunity to confirm or explicate these themes with as many people as it takes to feel confident in the plausibility and authenticity of subsequent analysis and interpretations (see Chapter 10 for further discussion of the plausibility of research findings).

Any research approach is underpinned by certain assumptions about the world and about how knowledge may be acquired. These assumptions 'have organizing effects on both the material gathered in research studies and on the way this material is represented as "data" or findings' (Cheek 1996, p. 492). Indeed, Holman (1993) observed that even 'the results of controlled [medical] experiments are often interpreted in accordance with the personal beliefs of the investigator' (p. 30). Because no development of a hypothesis or assessment of a research finding can occur without human interpretation (irrespective of the chosen methodology), it is pertinent to examine the assumptions that underpin qualitative approaches to research.

CHARACTERISTICS AND ASSUMPTIONS OF QUALITATIVE RESEARCH

Common to all qualitative theoretical perspectives are certain underlying assumptions:

- Human behaviour goes beyond what can be observed, incorporating subjective meanings, values and perceptions.
- Human behaviour, actions and ideas can only be understood in context, not separated from the physical, economic and sociocultural environments in which they function.
- People, including researchers (following any research methodology), perceive and interpret reality differently, based on the context of their past experiences; there are no 'objective' truths.

The research process and setting

Qualitative research is grounded in a concern with people's everyday realities, seeking to understand how people experience and make sense of their lives. Thus, the research is undertaken in a natural setting, such as a home, school or community clinic, rather than a research laboratory or 'controlled' environment.

The qualitative research process is both flexible and systematic, responding situationally to the research situation but following an overarching research plan. Qualitative research is often initiated in response to a clinical irritant or a foreshadowed problem: an issue, puzzle, or evident gap in understanding or knowledge that has arisen during the course of clinical practice or reviews of existing literature (see, for example, Chapter 3).

The role of the researcher: positioning and reflexivity

The researcher is recognized as being an integral part of the research process, shaping the collection of data and interpreting, explaining or describing human behaviour from the perspectives of those participating in the study. Engaging in an intellectual process through which the knowledge and experience of those under study is juxtaposed with the knowledge, sensitizing concepts and experience of the researcher, the outcome of the research is clearly a joint construction: both parties work together to generate the research findings. Acknowledging this fact, Karen Hammell explores issues of 'voice', the politics of representation and accountability to study participants in Chapter 6, suggesting that knowledge constructed jointly must be disseminated to the benefit of both parties in the research endeavour.

'Reflexivity' demands assessment of the influence of the investigator's background, perceptions and interests on the research process (Krefting 1991). It is recognized that the 'position' (gender, class, 'race', sexual orientation, age, religion, [dis]ability and other dimensions of social differentiation and of access to power) of the researcher will affect the research relationship and the nature of the data collected. Positioning is frequently regarded as problematic in qualitative research if there are significant discrepancies between the researcher and the researched in terms of these axes of differentiation; therefore as an integral part of the research process the researcher must analyse him or herself in the context of the research (Krefting 1991; see also Chapter 3). We will revisit the concepts of reflexivity and positionality in the final chapter of this book.

Shakespeare (1996) notes that the idea of the 'neutral researcher' is ultimately a fiction. He stresses that it is possible to be independent as a researcher, despite closeness to the project, but cautions against confusing independence with being 'neutral' or 'objective', as this is not possible for any researcher, following any methodology. In qualitative research this position is analysed rather than ignored.

Presentation of data

Qualitative research data are presented in narrative form, to preserve and represent the voices of the study participants (this will be noted in the following chapters). Thus, the written text of a piece of qualitative research will look different from the more familiar presentation of columns of numbers and tables of equations and statistics used in quantitative inquiry. The use of the transcribed voices of the study participants throughout the written report helps to re-present the participants' viewpoints.

Data analysis

Further, analysis of the data is often inductive and interpretive, that is reasoning from specific incidences and recurrent patterns within data is linked to general conclusions or principles. Although such 'thematic analysis' is commonly used by qualitative researchers (see, for example, Chapter 3), this is by no means the only way in which data may be analysed. Atkinson (1992) demonstrates how any analysis or written account of qualitative research must be understood to be just one of many possible interpretations or methods of documentation. He shows how the same set of data can be read and interpreted according to different analytical strategies. Acknowledging this reality, and seeking to avoid a relativistic position wherein 'one interpretation is as good as another' Harris (1996) suggests that researchers need to acknowledge that each analysis is but one of several possibilities, and thereby defend their own choice, based upon the purpose and nature of the research itself.

Qualitative research can also be utilized to explore the limits and build upon existing theories; and this will be further explored in Chapter 8.

THE CONGRUENCY OF QUALITATIVE RESEARCH METHODOLOGY WITH REHABILITATION

There are four issues of particular concern to occupational therapists and physical therapists that have resonance with qualitative research methodology.

Client-centred practice

First, there is the current focus upon client-centred practice: collaborative and partnership approaches to practice that encourage client autonomy, choice and control, and that respect clients' abilities and support their rights to enact those choices (Canadian Association of Occupational Therapists 1997). The ethics that inform a client-centred approach to practice include a regard for client values, support for both success and risk, facilitation of client-identified needs, and open communication with reciprocal exchange of information. Thus the philosophy underpinning client-centred practice is concerned with ensuring the meaningfulness of intervention, valuing the clients' knowledge, and respecting their life experiences.

Effective problem solving during rehabilitation requires an understanding of the client's perspective on what the problem is, yet much evidence suggests that client and professional perspectives differ in many critical areas (Corning 1999). For example, Abberley (1995) observed that occupational therapists are typically involved in a process of adjusting the client's view of reality to match their own (a process deemed 'educational'), yet examples in the literature suggest the futility of interventions based on therapists' priorities. It has been suggested that professional competence has two components. One dimension is a sound grasp of the techniques or formal knowledge of the profession: the other aspect is 'the ability to enter the patient's life-world so that the techniques are tailored to meet the patient's needs' (Crepeau 1991, p. 1024). Clearly, this is congruent with the philosophy informing qualitative research. Adopting a client-centred philosophy places the same emphasis upon understanding the client's perspective as does qualitative research. Recognition of the multiple realities – or experiences – of living means placing the same value upon the experiential knowledge of the client as on the theoretical knowledge of the therapist or researcher.

Community-based rehabilitation

Secondly, qualitative research is congruent with the contemporary emphasis upon community-based rehabilitation. Changing demographics, increasing longevity with chronic illnesses, political leanings toward care 'in the community', and professional recognition that the most effective interventions are those that occur in the context of the client's habitual environment have led to enhanced emphasis upon the deinstitutionalization of occupational therapy and physical therapy services. From this perspective, clients are viewed as inseparable from their context: family, friends, home, community and the larger physical, social, cultural, political, economic and historic circumstances that circumscribe their lives; thus the onus is upon the therapist or researcher to enter – and seek to understand – the dynamics of the client's environment, rather than the reverse (as is the situation in acute care and institutional settings). If rehabilitation is construed as the process of learning to live with a disability in the context of one's own environment, it could reasonably be proposed that this is the most appropriate context within which to frame our interventions.

Ethics

Thirdly, there is a clear congruence between the philosophy underpinning qualitative methodologies and that informing contemporary healthcare ethics. Until recently, the Hippocratic tradition dominated health care, such that patient preferences were set aside if they conflicted with the professional's view of what was in the patient's 'best interest'. Contemporary ethics propose that the competent client is the decision-maker, can refuse interventions and has the right to live at risk (although this right may be overruled if the desired intervention is likely to be futile or may be harmful to others). Fundamental to the notion of an autonomy-based ethic is the issue of informed consent. Thus, the philosophy of client-centred practice is not unique to occupational or physical therapy, nor is it an optional modus operandi. Rather, current biomedical ethics demand that the principles of client autonomy are respected. It is the issue of client autonomy – demanding respect for the values, beliefs, opinions and choices of the competent client (or surrogate) – that has particular relevance to both client-centred practice and to qualitative methodologies seeking to understand the perspectives of the client and the values that inform behaviour and motivations. In Chapter 7, Sue Forwell describes a study in which ethical issues influenced every stage of the research design: a study of undergraduate occupational therapy students undertaken by faculty researchers.

Quality of life

Finally, there is much current interest in 'measuring' the quality of life experienced by various client groups. Rehabilitation lore states that an increased level of physical function leads to enhanced quality of life. However, much research using quantitative methods suggests that, counter-intuitively, perceptions of quality of life do not correlate with level of function, degree of impairment, degree of disability or level of independence. Further, researchers have found that the two most popular measures of rehabilitation outcome – physical function and psychological adjustment – fail to correlate with each other. This raises the question: 'If quality of life is not determined by the severity of disability, what factors explain it?' In recognition of the impossibility of quantifying the inherently qualitative, the need to use qualitative research methods to assess 'quality' outcomes would appear to be self-evident.

QUALITATIVE RESEARCH: THE FIT WITH OCCUPATIONAL AND PHYSICAL THERAPIES

Physical therapists and occupational therapists need to inform their practice through a deep understanding of their clients' perspectives. Both groups of professionals provide interventions to human beings – not nerves, muscles or superegos (Yerxa 1991) – and so both research and clinical practice must seek to elicit relevant knowledge and understanding. The professions recognize that human beings interact with their environments in a complex dynamic; therefore, research methods should be utilized that will address this interaction.

There is increasing recognition that people endow their lives, experiences and activities with meaning, influenced by a personal equation of language, culture, history and spiritual values. Clients may share a diagnosis with other clients, but interventions must be applicable to the unique environment, life stage and goals of each individual. The diversity of meanings about disability that people hold and the place disability assumes within individual biographies need to be considered in research and practice. Again, there is a clear fit between qualitative research methodology and contemporary rehabilitation practice, providing a means by which to attain a holistic view of the individual in context.

Rehabilitation practitioners often claim to be involved in seeking to enhance their clients' 'quality of life'. A persuasive argument can be made that quality of life outcomes can only be ascertained by understanding the value that clients place upon their subjective experiences of living (Peters 1996): this demands qualitative modes of inquiry. Jensen (1989) argued that qualitative methods have special relevance for physical therapy, providing researchers with the tools to examine both complex environments and human behaviour. Qualitative methods 'are well suited to studying the complex, multi-dimensional environments present in physical therapy practice and education' (Jensen 1989, p. 492). Similarly, Yerxa (1991) claimed that occupational therapists need to seek ways of knowing that are different from the statistical methods of the physical sciences and which reflect the humanistic values of the profession. Yerxa proposes that 'qualitative research approaches have a goodness of fit with finding out what is worth knowing for occupational therapists' (p. 200).

CONTRIBUTIONS OF QUALITATIVE RESEARCH TO THEORETICAL DEVELOPMENT

Theory, although understated (or even unstated) is what guides all clinical practice and every research inquiry: informing what we believe

should be done in various situations. Thus, all research or systematic evaluation of clinical practice and outcomes may be viewed as supporting or contesting existing theoretical paradigms.

Neither of the academic disciplines of physical therapy or occupational therapy has benefited from extensive or rigorous research to inform the development of their unique theoretical bases, reflecting, in part, the historic dearth of scholars holding doctoral degrees in either. Fortunately, this situation is now changing and it is therefore timely to consider our theoretical foundations and whether we can support our beliefs. Does our knowledge base reflect our assumptions, ethics and philosophy of practice? What else do we need to know? How can we address theory most effectively? Qualitative research can be useful in several ways to develop and evaluate theory.

Whereas quantitative research is approached with a theory already to hand for which a specific hypothesis is to be tested, qualitative research is a cyclical process wherein data is collected and analysed, and patterns and themes identified. Concurrently, the researcher compares emerging ideas and data with various theoretical concepts that might explain or account for the data, with additional data being sought to further explicate theory (Krefting 1989). In this way qualitative data can be used to reaffirm, revise or expand a particular theoretical framework (Shepard et al 1993).

By enabling the identification of conceptual links within the data and the subsequent development of conceptual frameworks, qualitative research may constitute a catalyst for conceptualization, with hypotheses following from the data rather than preceding it (as in traditional, quantitative studies; Krefting 1989). Box 1.1 highlights some of the ways in which qualitative research may contribute to the theories and knowledge that underpin our professions.

CONCLUSION

Crucial to the development of the academic disciplines of occupational therapy and

---

> **Box 1.1** Contributions to theory: a multidimensional role
>
> ◆ Qualitative research is particularly useful in generating new research questions by exposing inconsistencies in – or limits to – current knowledge and theories.
> ◆ Qualitative inquiry enables the identification of formerly unrecognized relationships among elements of a phenomenon (Shepard et al 1993, Peters 1996).
> ◆ This identification may thereafter provide a foundation for the generation of new hypotheses and further (perhaps quantitative) investigation (Krefting 1989, Shepard et al 1993, Peters 1996). Thus, qualitative and quantitative methodologies may be complementary.
> ◆ Qualitative data enable researchers to use information gleaned from data analysis to reaffirm, contest or revise theory, thereby determining the conditions under which theory may be supported (Shepard et al 1993).
> ◆ Because qualitative researchers do not begin with specific hypotheses they are less likely to overlook phenomena that do not fit their prior expectations (Krefting 1989). Used in concert with quantitative methods, qualitative methods thus increase our ability to understand and explain 'outliers', or atypical responses (Krefting 1991).

physical therapy is recognition that the term 'research' does not, by default, imply a particular or preferred approach to the acquisition of knowledge. No single approach is adequate to the task of exploring the complexity of human experience or behaviour (Peters 1996).

Yerxa (1987, p. 415) observed that: 'Research is a systematic way of observing some aspect of the world and describing it so that it can be better understood'. Central to our argument throughout this book is the position that research methodologies should be selected solely on the basis of their fit with the nature of the problem to be investigated, enabling us to better understand.

It may be argued that both our academic disciplines have been the poorer for our traditional tendency to try to emulate the methodologies of the physical sciences, and thereafter to explore only those questions that can usefully be addressed via this approach. Frequently this has led our researchers to contribute to the knowledge bases of other

disciplines, such as physiology, psychology or kinesiology, rather than to our own, thereby perpetuating the study of minds or muscles rather than of human beings.

Both occupational therapy and physical therapy – as evolving, dynamic academic disciplines – require knowledge bases grounded on an understanding of how human beings adapt to changing internal and external conditions that affect their capacity to move and act in and on their environments, through time and in changing circumstances. Rather than borrowing research techniques and objects of inquiry more appropriate to incompatible academic fields of study (such as physics), we should ask: 'What is worth knowing in our own disciplines and what research tools are most appropriate in this endeavour?' The following chapters aim to demonstrate the usefulness of qualitative research methods to the evolving knowledge bases of our disciplines by drawing on examples of research studies undertaken by ourselves and our colleagues.

REFERENCES

Abberley P 1995 Disabling ideology in health and welfare – the case of occupational therapy. Disability and Society 10:221–232

Atkinson P 1992 The ethnography of a medical setting: reading, writing, and rhetoric. Qualitative Health Research 2(4):451–474

Barnes C 1992 Qualitative research: valuable or irrelevant? Disability, Handicap and Society 7(2):115–124

Bogdan RC Biklen SK 1998 Qualitative research for education: an introduction to theory and methods, 3rd edn. Allyn & Bacon, Boston

Canadian Association of Occupational Therapists 1997 Enabling occupation. An occupational therapy perspective. Canadian Association of Occupational Therapists, Ottawa

Cancian FM 1992 Feminist science: methodologies that challenge inequality. Gender and Society 6(4):623–642

Carpenter C 1997 Conducting qualitative research in physiotherapy: a methodological example. Physiotherapy 83(10):547–552

Cheek J 1996 Taking a view: qualitative research as representation. Qualitative Health Research 6(4):492–505

Corning DJ 1999 The missing perspective on client-centred care. Occupational Therapy Now Jan-Feb:8–10

Crepeau EB 1991 Achieving intersubjective understanding: examples from an occupational therapy treatment session. American Journal of Occupational Therapy 45:1016–1025

Creswell J 1998 Qualitative inquiry and research design: choosing among *five* traditions. Sage, Thousand Oaks

Field PA, Morse JM 1985 Nursing research. The application of qualitative methods. Chapman & Hall, London

Harris A 1996 Responsibility and advocacy: representing young women. In: Wilkinson S, Kitzinger C (eds) Representing the other. Sage, London, pp 152–155

Hasselkus BR 1991 Qualitative research: not another orthodoxy. Occupational Journal of Research 11(1):3–7

Holman HR 1993 Qualitative inquiry in medical research. Journal of Clinical Epidemiology 46(1):29–36

Jensen GM 1989 Qualitative methods in physical therapy research: a form of disciplined inquiry. Physical Therapy 69:492–500

Keysor JJ, Sparling JW, Riegger-Krugh C 1998 The experience of knee arthritis in athletic young and middle-aged adults: an heuristic study. Arthritis Care and Research 11(4):261–270

Krefting L 1989 Disability ethnography: a methodological approach for occupational therapy research. Canadian Journal of Occupational Therapy 56(2):61–66

Krefting L 1991 Rigor in qualitative research: the assessment of trustworthiness. American Journal of Occupational Therapy 45(3):214–222

Marcus GE, Fischer MMJ 1986 Anthropology as cultural critique. An experimental moment in the human sciences. University of Chicago Press, Chicago

Peters DJ 1996 Qualitative inquiry. Expanding rehabilitation medicine's research repertoire: a commentary. American Journal of Physical Medicine and Rehabilitation 75(2):144–148

Shakespeare T 1996 Rules of engagement: doing disability research. Disability and Society 11(1):115–119

Shepard KF, Jensen GM, Schmoll BJ, Hack LM, Gwyer J 1993 Alternative approaches to research in physical therapy: positivism and phenomenology. Physical Therapy 73:88–97

Spencer J, Krefting L, Mattingly C 1993 Incorporation of ethnographic methods in occupational therapy assessment. American Journal of Occupational Therapy 47(4):303–309

Yerxa EJ 1987 Research: the key to the development of occupational therapy as an academic discipline. American Journal of Occupational Therapy 41(7):415–419

Yerxa EJ 1991 Seeking a relevant, ethical, and realistic way of knowing for occupational therapy. American Journal of Occupational Therapy 45(3):199–204

FURTHER READING

Hammersley M, Atkinson P 1995 Ethnography: principles in practice, 2nd edn. Routledge, London

Spencer J 1993 The usefulness of qualitative methods in rehabilitation: issues of meaning, of context, and of change. Archives of Physical Medicine and Rehabilitation 74:119–126

2

Choosing the methodology to explore the research

Lyn Jongbloed

KEY POINTS
qualitative and quantitative research methodologies: characteristics, underlying assumptions and complementarity of uses; multiple sclerosis

OVERVIEW

The purpose of this chapter is to discuss the paradigm upon which qualitative research is based, and to distinguish it from quantitative research. A study of women with multiple sclerosis (MS) is used to illustrate how the two methodologies differ and how they can be combined.

TWO RESEARCH PARADIGMS

Research paradigms encompass beliefs about ways of obtaining knowledge (Lincoln & Guba 1985). The two main research paradigms used in occupational therapy and physical therapy are quantitative and qualitative. These differ in terms of philosophical tradition, the form of reasoning used and ways of obtaining knowledge (DePoy & Gitlin 1994). Table 2.1 identifies these differences.

Table 2.1   Assumptions of qualitative and quantitative approaches (adapted from Domholdt (1993) Table 9-2, with permission)

Assumption	Qualitative	Quantitative
Epistemology	Multiple realities	Single objective reality
Purpose	Reveal complexity Identify meanings	Explain Predict
Relationship between researcher and subject	Interdependent	Independent
Values	Value bound	Value free
Cause-and-effect relationships	Non-causal	Causal
Generalizability of findings	Situation specific Theoretical constructs may be generalized to other samples, settings, situations	Desirable

The qualitative approach

The qualitative paradigm assumes that the world consists of many constructed realities, i.e. the meanings that people assign to events form an integral part of those events. The world, and people's experiences of that world, cannot be separated. Individual perceptions of the world therefore form the basis of knowledge (Guba 1990). In terms of chronic illness, the focus is on the subjective experience of living with that illness. The purpose of research is to develop an understanding of the perspectives of people in such a setting, and to develop theory. The researcher and the subject are viewed as interdependent, and the research process alters both the subject and the researcher. Research is value laden, and this is evidenced in how questions are asked and findings interpreted. It is impossible to separate causes from effects: the researcher therefore aims to describe and interpret events, rather than to verify causes and effects; the knowledge that is produced relates to a specific time and place. The goal is an in-depth understanding of a particular setting, rather

than a generalization of findings to other people and settings (Domholdt 1993), although theoretical concepts that are developed may be applicable to other settings.

The quantitative approach

The quantitative paradigm assumes that there is a single objective reality, and that it is possible to know this reality outside oneself (Guba 1990). The purpose of research is therefore to explain and predict aspects of reality. The researcher and the subjects should be independent. Research is viewed as value free. Because the research is considered controlled and objective, the investigator's ideas are not seen as influencing it. Cause and effect can be ascertained, and this is done by manipulating an independent variable and observing its effect on a dependent variable. It is considered desirable that research be conducted in such a way that findings are generalizable to other people, settings and times (Domholdt 1993).

USE OF QUALITATIVE AND QUANTITATIVE APPROACHES IN A STUDY

Qualitative and quantitative research approaches are affected in fundamental ways by these different assumptions. I will use a study of women with multiple sclerosis (MS) (conducted with Isabel Dyck) to illustrate how the assumptions underlying each paradigm influence its methods. This research collaboration capitalized on Isabel Dyck's expertise and knowledge in using qualitative research, and my background in quantitative research, to address questions related to women and disability. In the process we came to appreciate how much we could learn from each other.

The purpose of the study was to investigate the work experiences of women with MS, which has an unpredictable cause, no cure and a variety of symptoms. A literature search indicated that most research had adopted an individualistic approach to explain the employment status of those with MS, focusing on demographic and disease characteristics and specific workplace features. Little research had drawn on the workplace experiences of women with disabilities from their perspectives. Even less had attempted to incorporate the influence of broad societal relations and economic processes in understanding the disability experience. Our study adopted a sociopolitical model of disability (Hahn 1986, Jongbloed & Crichton 1990) which emphasizes the social, cultural, economic and political influences on disability. We aimed to explore (1) the barriers to paid employment that women with MS experience; (2) the resources (both formal and informal) that women draw on in attempting to manage disability in the workplace; (3) the adjustments they make in both wage and domestic work in response to changes accompanying the course of the disease; and (4) the nature of constraints shaping their responses.

Our study employed both qualitative and quantitative approaches. Because little was known about the workplace experiences of women with MS from their point of view, we used qualitative methods (defined in Chapter 1) to identify, describe and analyse those experiences. Semi-structured, in-depth interviews explored various aspects of the lives of two groups of women with MS who had been employed at the time of diagnosis, namely those who were still employed and those no longer employed.

The findings of the qualitative phase stood alone in providing conceptual development and a descriptive account of the experiences of women with MS. An in-depth understanding of issues important to women with MS, obtained from the qualitative phase, also assisted us in the formulation of hypotheses to be tested on a large group of women in the quantitative phase and in the development of questions to be included in the mail questionnaire sent to these women.

Each research approach is presented below in terms of relationship to theory, design, subject selection, setting, instruments, nature of the data and data analysis. Table 2.2 summarizes the two approaches in terms of these dimensions.

Table 2.2 Comparison of qualitative and quantitative methods

Method	Qualitative	Quantitative
Relationship to theory	Theory generation Inductive	Theory verification Deductive
Design	Flexible: responsive to research situation	Structured Predetermined
Subject selection	Purposive Non-representative	Probability sampling
Setting	Natural	Controlled
Instruments	Researcher Tape/video recorder	Instruments should be reliable and valid
Nature of data	Narratives of subjects Field notes Documents	Scores on standardized scales
Data analysis	Ongoing (cyclical) Coding, sorting	Statistical analysis at the end of data collection

Qualitative phase of research project

Relationship to theory

Qualitative research aims to describe the experiences of people in particular settings and to understand their perspectives. Its purpose is also to develop hypotheses, concepts and theory. We focused our research on people's daily lives as carried out in the communities where they live and work, for it is there that the consequences of disability acquire meaning (Anderson & Bury 1988). Our goal was to understand what strategies women with MS employ in dealing with their disability in the workplace, what adjustments they make at home and work in response to changes in their disease, and how the work, home and policy environments enable or constrain them. With unemployed women with MS, the objective was to describe how they manage the physical, social and economic consequences of their illness. We thereafter developed hypotheses to be tested in the quantitative phase of the project.

Design

Qualitative research designs are flexible and may evolve throughout the study. A general phenomenon of interest is identified and more specific questions emerge in the process of conducting the research (DePoy & Gitlin 1994). In the process of interviewing women with MS, it became clear that the visibility/invisibility of symptoms was important, as were decisions regarding the disclosure of symptoms to others, and so these concepts were included in later interviews.

Participant selection

In qualitative research the researcher selects people who are likely to increase understanding of the research topic. The sample may be either purposive or convenience. We chose people who attended the MS clinic or who belonged to a local MS Society, and who had been employed at the time of diagnosis, as they would be informed about the consequences of MS in relation to workforce participation.

   The number of participants is not determined in advance. The sample needs to be broad enough to encompass some variety and variability. Actual sample size is determined by the quality and completeness of the information collected. When repetitive information is obtained, this is an indication that saturation has been achieved (DePoy & Gitlin 1994). We had planned to interview approximately 40 people, but it was not until we had interviewed more than 60 that we felt satisfied with the quality and completeness of our information.

Researcher's relationship with participants

The researcher and the participant are engaged in a collaborative relationship and both are changed by the research process (Reinharz 1992). We established rapport, developed trust and empathized with the women, and learned a great deal from them. They, in turn, appeared to value our interest in listening to their stories.

Setting

Qualitative research focuses on ordinary events in natural settings. The researcher sees and interacts with the individual in his or her own context. We learned a great deal about women's lives by talking to them in their home or work environments.

Instrument

The researcher is the primary instrument of data collection. Because the purpose of the research is to reveal the complexities of many different perspectives, the investigator needs to be an engaged, thoughtful, instrument (Domholdt 1993). In our study, the two investigators and the research assistant interviewed participants, made observations, reviewed transcripts of interviews, conceptualized and articulated emerging themes, identified new issues to be raised with future participants and reviewed data in terms of existing knowledge.

Nature of data

Data collected in qualitative research are descriptive and include the words of subjects, expressing feelings and ideas, as well as observation and personal or official documents.

   Interviews can vary in terms of degree of structure. They may be directed by informants, in which case the interviewer does not have prearranged questions and the goal is that the informants provide the important data (Krefting 1989). Semi-structured interviews can also be used: here the researcher presents the study purpose and starts with a broad general question, such as: 'Can you tell me what life has been like for you since you were diagnosed with multiple sclerosis?' Other questions emerge as the participant responds to this initial query (DePoy & Gitlin 1994).

   In our study we conducted semi-structured, in-depth interviews to explore different aspects of women's lives, including work experiences, income issues, personal relationships and illness management strategies. Although some questions were asked of all participants, the participants themselves controlled the direction of the interviews to some extent. Interviews were tape-recorded and then transcribed on to a computer verbatim to preserve the language of the participants. For example, one unemployed woman described how her activities were curtailed by lack of income: 'On social assistance, you're on the poverty line. I'm just existing. If I was working, I'd be able to visit and go and do a few things. This way I can do nothing. I don't even have the bus fare, you know.'

Review of documents constitutes another qualitative research strategy. This involves reviewing relevant legislation as well as written materials such as medical records, letters or diaries. Data analysis and review of the academic literature to see how research findings fit with existing knowledge form an ongoing circular process (Krefting 1989). We reviewed legislation and policies related to people with disabilities in the areas of income, employment, housing, transportation and assistance at home. We also examined the literature on women's employment, women and disabilities, as well as social science literature on the ways in which the social, economic, cultural and political environments shape people's daily lives.

Data analysis

Data analysis involves reading notes and transcripts of interviews, identifying themes, and then incorporating those themes into the next stage of data collection. Data collection and analysis are therefore interdependent. The analysis is inductive, in that themes and concepts emerge from the data. The researcher then develops linkages between various parts of the data, comparing linkages/generalizations with existing theoretical concepts (Miles & Huberman 1994). Issues concerning reliability and validity are addressed through systematic recording of the research process, triangulation through the use of different types of data collection, and through a team approach to data analysis, as well as logical consistency in

interpretation (DePoy & Gitlin 1994). These issues will be discussed in more detail in Chapter 10.

The two investigators and the research assistant read the transcripts of the first 10 interviews and found that many women talked about particular issues, including the following: employment, disclosure, income issues, household work organization, relationships, lifestyle/activity changes, strategies for coping with MS, support and managing/experiencing the environment. These themes then shaped future interviews in that we ensured that relevant issues were raised with each participant.

We identified and discussed emerging themes from the interviews and then organized the themes into categories. The three team members coded each transcript independently. Final coding of the data occurred during team meetings, when any inconsistencies in coding were discussed and resolved. We generated both descriptive and analytical accounts of significant relationships and processes that shaped people's experiences and integrated these with existing theoretical constructs. Although the data analysis included reaching a consensus on the themes and concepts emerging from the data, it was informed by the different perspectives and theoretical interests of the two researchers. One investigator used concepts of the political and economic environment to examine how the structuring of disability benefit programmes shapes the individual experience of disability (Jongbloed 1998). She also examined the social context framing the decisions of women with MS to remain employed or to leave employment (Jongbloed 1996).

The other investigator used geographical concepts of space and place to explore the everyday lives of unemployed women with MS to reveal the complex interweaving of space, physical impairment and gender in how they experience place (Dyck 1995). The home became these women's primary activity space, as indicated by this comment: 'Your home environment changes quite a bit. You're constantly around it … it has to be your whole resource.' This is expressed in the concept we termed 'shrinking social and geographical worlds'. Residential relocation occurred for many women, but this was constrained by marital status, income and financial assets. Non-married women were more likely to be constrained by costs in terms of choice of housing. The women experienced increased dependence on others for self-care and house-hold tasks; and wider social, economic and political forces intruded into their private space as they were assessed for their eligibility for home care and homemaker services, and then had service providers penetrate their home environment (Dyck 1995). Dyck (1999) also examined issues related to disclosure of the diagnosis in the workplace, and the strategies women used to conceal their disabilities.

Qualitative analysis is concerned with the careful definition of concepts and the development of theoretical constructs that provide the basis for generalization to other samples, settings and situations (Hammersley & Atkinson 1995). So, for example, the concept of shrinking geographical and social worlds found among unemployed women with MS may also apply to those with other disabilities.

Quantitative phase of research project

Relationship to theory

The purpose of quantitative research is to describe, explain or predict phenomena. Research questions are developed from existing theory and the research tests various aspects of theory. In our quantitative study there were particular questions we wished to answer. We wanted to find out what distinguishes women who remained employed from those who were no longer employed in terms of demographics, disease, employment conditions and other factors. For those still employed, we wished to determine what kinds of difficulties women with MS experienced at work, and what conditions at work and outside work enabled

people to continue employment. For those no longer employed, the objective was to identify the primary reasons given by women for leaving their last place of employment. We also wanted to assess the typicality of the case material found in the qualitative phase. Past research on employment among people with MS and other disabilities informed our research questions related to disease and demographic variables, and the social science literature challenged us to examine the contexts that shaped women's decisions. The qualitative phase of the research project also alerted us to issues that women identified as being important factors affecting their employment status, and which had not previously been identified in research using quantitative designs.

Design

Quantitative designs are structured and determined before data collection and analysis begin. Quantitative research can be classified as non-experimental, quasi-experimental and experimental (Domholdt 1993). Our research was non-experimental, as it did not involve the manipulation of an independent variable. We conducted a mail survey of women with MS who had been employed at the time of diagnosis. Our objectives were to document how MS had affected women in paid employment, how they coped, and what factors in their environment (e.g. employers, flexible schedules, supportive family members) contributed to their decisions to continue or discontinue employment. Questions to be asked were informed by the qualitative study and identified in advance. The way in which data would be analysed was also decided prior to data collection.

Subject selection

The researcher identifies the characteristics of the population to be studied and then selects a sample of that group for the study. Ways of sampling have been developed which ensure that the sample accurately represents the population, and findings can be generalized to the population from which they are drawn. The population for our quantitative study was all women with a definite diagnosis of multiple sclerosis, aged 19–60, who had attended the MS clinic at the University of British Columbia. We mailed questionnaires to all 864 women who fitted these inclusion criteria. Our population and sample were thus identical, but because we obtained our subjects from a particular medical setting, we could not generalize findings beyond this population.

Researcher's relationship with subjects

Because the objectivity of the researcher is valued, the relationship between the quantitative researcher and the subjects is detached. It is viewed as important that the researcher should not influence the data through involvement with subjects (Bailey 1991). We conducted a mail survey and thus had no contact with subjects.

Setting

The quantitative paradigm emphasizes controlling extraneous factors that might influence research findings. Thus a controlled environment, or a laboratory, is frequently the site of research. In our quantitative study the setting was not controlled.

Instruments

Data collection instruments may be scales, tests, questionnaires or hardware (Bailey 1991) which are deemed to be both reliable and valid. In our study the subjects completed a structured questionnaire. Their responses to questions were controlled, in that they had to select from pre-established categories.

Type of data

The data collected are usually structured, quantifiable and objective (DePoy & Gitlin 1994). In our quantitative study, participants were asked to choose one of several predetermined

responses to each question. Each response on the questionnaire was converted into numerical form so that it could be analysed statistically.

Data analysis

Data are analysed at the end of data collection. Analysis is usually statistical, and can be completed quite rapidly. We compared employed women with unemployed women in terms of factors such as age, education, degree of disability, and job title when diagnosed with MS, and identified where there were statistically significant differences. We also identified which employment conditions were identified most frequently by women as enabling them to continue to work, as well as the main reasons given by women for leaving their last place of employment.

The findings of quantitative research provide answers to research questions posed at the beginning of the study (Domholdt 1993). Our study findings reported that women currently employed were statistically significantly younger, had more education, and were less disabled than those not currently employed. The most important employment conditions allowing people to continue to work were the ability to take sick time when needed (identified by 74%); having an understanding employer (identified by 60%); having understanding colleagues (identified by 63%); and flexible work hours (identified by 48%).

Integrating qualitative and quantitative approaches

Some researchers view the two research paradigms as incompatible because the assumptions and ideas upon which they are based are fundamentally different. They argue that adopting the assumptions of one paradigm means letting go of the assumptions of the other (Lincoln & Guba 1985). A more moderate view holds that the assumptions underlying each paradigm are relative, not absolute, and that qualitative and quantitative designs can be combined in three ways. First, qualitative and quantitative methods may be used to increase understanding about a particular issue. Second, one primary framework (qualitative or quantitative) may be used, but strategies from the other framework may be borrowed. Third, the frameworks of the two different paradigms may be used within a single research project to address different questions (DePoy & Gitlin 1994). Leininger (1985) stresses the importance of determining the reasons for combining or not combining the two methods. Our project utilized qualitative and quantitative approaches. The findings of the qualitative phase of the study stood alone in providing both a descriptive account and theoretical development of the experience of work for women who were employed, and the shrinking worlds experienced by many women who were no longer employed. It showed, for example, that the home and work contexts in which each individual functioned influenced her decisions regarding continuing or leaving employment. In many cases the interaction between an individual's symptoms and her job demands made it impossible to continue work. For example, the work of a registered nurse and a hairdresser is physically demanding. Several women found that their symptoms were such that they could no longer continue working. A hairdresser commented: 'I only worked for about another three months because I couldn't stand very long, and the vibrations bothered my left hand. And of course when you're hairdressing you have to hold a blow dryer in your left hand.'

In some instances employers adjusted work requirements to allow the person to continue work; this usually occurred in situations where the person had specialized education and a good track record in the organization. For example, a lawyer who felt she could not continue as a full-time partner in the firm, nor practise law part-time, was provided with a specially created part-time job within the firm, involving literature searches.

These in-depth studies of the lives of individual women helped us to understand the quantitative finding that education was a predictor of employment status: employers made little effort to adapt the work situation to the needs of less educated employees because they were seen as being more dispensable than those with more education. The findings of the qualitative phase were also integral to the quantitative phase in (1) clarifying questions to be posed in a mail questionnaire to a large group of women, and (2) enhancing the quality of the questions included in the questionnaire, as these were formulated from the issues identified by women with MS. Findings from the qualitative study alerted us to the importance of the social environment at work (i.e. flexible schedules, supportive employers and colleagues) in terms of enabling women to continue working. We were thus able to include questions about this in the mail questionnaire; and quantitative findings confirmed our suspicion that it was indeed an important factor for a large number of women. Thus concepts, ideas and hypotheses developed in the qualitative study were tested on a large number of subjects in the quantitative phase of the study; and findings from the quantitative study could be generalized to all women with MS who had attended that MS clinic.

CONCLUSION

Very different beliefs underlie the two main research paradigms used in occupational therapy and physical therapy. The dominant paradigm remains the quantitative, in which the goal of research is to explain or predict relationships between variables and to verify theory. The qualitative paradigm aims to enhance understanding of multiple perspectives of reality, and to develop theory. Both paradigms can be used within a single study to answer different questions or different parts of the same research question.

Acknowledgements

I wish to thank the women with MS who participated in the study referred to in this chapter. The research was funded by grants from the BC Health Research Foundation and the Social Sciences and Humanities Research Council. The principal investigator of the study was Isabel Dyck, School of Rehabilitation Sciences, University of British Columbia; and the research assistant was Bobbi Bagshaw.

REFERENCES

Anderson R, Bury M 1988 Living with chronic illness: the experiences of patients and their families. Unwin Hyman, London

Bailey D 1991 Research for the health professional: a practical guide. FA Davis, Philadelphia

DePoy E, Gitlin L 1994 Introduction to research: multiple strategies for health and human services. Mosby, Toronto

Domholdt E 1993 Physical therapy research: principles and applications. WB Saunders, Toronto

Dyck I 1995 Hidden geographies: the changing lifeworlds of women with multiple sclerosis. Social Science and Medicine 40(3):307–320

Dyck I 1998 Women with disabilities and everyday geographies: home space and the contested body. In: Kearns RA, Gesler WM (eds) Putting health into place: landscape, identity and well being. Syracuse Press, Syracuse, pp 102–119

Dyck I 1999 Body troubles: women, the workplace and negotiations of a disabled identity. In: Butler R, Parr H (eds) Mind and body spaces: geographies of disability, illness and impairments. Routledge, London (in press)

Guba EG 1990 Carrying on the dialogue. In: Guba EG (ed) The paradigm dialogue. Sage, Newbury Park, California, pp 368–378

Hahn H 1986 Public support for rehabilitation programs: the analysis of US disability policy. Disability, Handicap and Society 1:121–137

Hammersley M, Atkinson P 1995 Ethnography: principles in practice, 2nd edn. Routledge, London

Jongbloed L 1996 Factors influencing employment status of women with multiple sclerosis. Canadian Journal of Rehabilitation 9(4):213–222

Jongbloed L 1998 Disability income: the experiences of women with multiple sclerosis. Canadian Journal of Occupational Therapy 65(4):193–201

Jongbloed L, Crichton A 1990 A new definition of disability: implications for rehabilitation practice and social policy. Canadian Journal of Occupational Therapy 57(1):32–38

Krefting L 1989 Disability ethnography: a methodological approach for occupational therapy research. Canadian Journal of Occupational Therapy 56(2):61–66

Leininger M 1985 Nature, rationale and importance of qualitative research methods in nursing. In: Leininger M (ed) Qualitative research: methods in nursing. Grune and Stratton, Orlando, Florida, pp 1–26

Lincoln Y, Guba E 1985 Naturalistic inquiry. Sage, Newbury Park, California

Miles M, Huberman A 1994 Qualitative data analysis: an expanded sourcebook, 2nd edn. Sage, Thousand Oaks, California

Reinharz S 1992 Feminist methods in social research. Oxford University Press, New York

FURTHER READING

Carpenter C 1994 The experience of spinal cord injury: the individual's perspective – implications for rehabilitation practice. Physical Therapy 74(7):614–629

Helfrich C, Kielhofner G, Mattingly C 1994 Volition as narrative: understanding motivation in chronic illness. American Journal of Occupational Therapy 48(11):1006–1013

McCuaig M, Frank G 1991 The able self: adaptive patterns and choices in independent living for a person with cerebral palsy. American Journal of Occupational Therapy 45(3):224–234

Yerxa E 1991 Seeking a relevant, ethical and realistic way of knowing for occupational therapy. American Journal of Occupational Therapy 45(3):199–204

3

Exploring the lived experience of disability

Chris Carpenter

KEY POINTS

relationship between research question and choice of methodology; foreshadowed problem; participant sampling; researcher role; impact of research process on researcher; ethnographic semi-structured interviews; data analysis; spinal cord injury

CHAPTER CONTENTS

OVERVIEW

This chapter describes a study which explored individual perceptions of the experience of traumatic spinal cord injury, and focuses on the central role I played, as the researcher, in collecting and analysing the data, and interacting with the study participants. The impact of the research process in raising my awareness of the attitudes, assumptions and preconceptions I held about disability will be explored, and suggestions offered about the contributions this type of study can make to rehabilitation practice.

RESEARCH QUESTIONS IN REHABILITATION

Research in spinal cord injury rehabilitation has focused primarily on issues concerning the provision of care and on treatment intervention outcome measures. This focus has served the needs of specific disciplines and contributed to programme development in rehabilitation. However, the input of those who have sustained injuries resulting in disability has not been solicited in a consistent or systematic way. It is therefore hardly surprising that clinical research in the area of spinal cord injury rehabilitation conducted by physical therapists has focused primarily on physical outcomes related to, for example, gait training, wheelchair management, muscle strength or respiratory function. The choice of research methodology is directed by the questions being raised in clinical practice and, traditionally, questions in rehabilitation about the efficacy of care and functional outcomes have been addressed using a quantitative research approach. However, some questions arising from clinical practice and the observation of clients clearly cannot be answered using a quantitative approach. For example:

- What does success in learning to live with disability mean to persons who have sustained a traumatic injury?
- How are these definitions of success consistent or inconsistent with the goals of therapy in the rehabilitation setting?
- What are the long-term consequences of living with a spinal cord injury?
- What do clients with a spinal cord injury need to know to better prepare them for the ageing process?

The qualitative tradition offers an alternative approach to clinical research when the questions raised relate to:

- a client's perspective
- the meanings made by an individual of an experience of a particular phenomenon
- the impact of contextual factors on the rehabilitation process
- the complexity or power dynamics of interactions.

THE STUDY

The clinical dilemma or 'foreshadowed problem'

The clinical dilemma or 'foreshadowed problem' (Hammersley & Atkinson 1995) that triggered

this study arose from many years of clinical practice as a physical therapist in spinal cord injury rehabilitation. According to Hammersley and Atkinson (1995), these 'generalized foreshadowed problems' are identified and thereafter refined by 'analytic reflection', which is facilitated by observation and theoretical reading. Through my involvement with a newly established fertility clinic for individuals with spinal cord injury, I had the unique opportunity to talk with, and learn from, individuals who were getting on with their lives, and who were many years post injury. For these individuals, their visit to the clinic was the first time they had returned to the rehabilitation centre since their discharge post injury. My conversations with these 'old hands', as they called themselves, revealed a discrepancy between the perception of spinal cord injury and its consequences held by myself and my colleagues, and that held by those who experience the injury over time. These conversations suggested that their individual responses to the injury could be more effectively understood in the light of a significant life event, defined by Dohrenwend and Dohrenwend (1974) as a life event that is 'indicative of, or requires a significant change in, the ongoing life pattern of the individual' (p. 2). This definition emphasizes the change from an existing steady state but does not categorize the event as inherently positive or negative: such an interpretation can only be made by an individual in relation to the meaning attributed to the event. It was from these encounters and the new insights I was gaining that this study evolved.

Choice of methodology

I was interested in answering the question: 'What is the experience of spinal cord injury like for you personally?' This interest in individual reality lends itself to the methodology known as phenomenology, and involves some form of interpretation on the part of both the participant and the researcher. Phenomenology was the qualitative approach chosen for this study because the aim was to describe perceptions of lived experience rather than to categorize, explain or define it, and the research question arose from a desire to understand behaviour from an individual's frame of reference and social context. In this study the phenomenon to be explored was the individual experience of traumatic spinal cord injury over time.

Research participants

Because the focus in phenomenological research is on the meanings *individuals* give to a particular experience, the researcher has to identify a sample of people who will be able to participate because they have personal experience of the phenomenon under study (Clifford 1997). For the purposes of this study, initial access to a network of potential participants was gained through the sponsorship offered by a personal acquaintance, himself a quadriplegic (tetraplegic), who was working as a social worker with a peer support group. His explanation of the study to the group resulted in three people volunteering to be involved. The participant selection criteria were simply that they were *self*-defined as successful or 'back on track' in their lives, and had sustained a complete spinal cord injury 3–5 years ago. Because of the in-depth nature of qualitative research many studies require small select samples, and specific sampling methods have been developed for this approach (Clifford 1997). The participant sampling technique used in this study is described as 'snowball sampling', whereby the initial participants are asked to recommend others whom they would define in a similar way. In this manner a total of 12 individuals became involved (Table 3.1) and I was able to focus on their self-definitions, rather than on my own opinions or judgements. All the participants were provided with a full written explanation of the research project and what was involved for them, and each signed a consent form. However, because the qualitative research process – data collection and analysis – is one of discovery, I undertook to provide further explanations as necessary during and after the interviews, and the participants remained free to withdraw at any stage and to refuse to answer any questions.

Table 3.1 Description of individuals who participated in the research study

Name*	Age	Injury (all complete)	Years post injury at time of interview	Interests
Tricia	21	Cervical	3	Attending college
William	39	Thoracic	4	Metalwork Wheelchair racing
Larry	28	Thoracic	3	Using newly acquired accounting qualifications
Malcolm	31	Cervical	4	Professional music production
Peter	39	Thoracic	4	Competitive tennis
Randy	35	Cervical	5	Using computer skills
Brian	32	Cervical	5	Planning his wedding
Dirk	35	Cervical	5	His relationship with partner and sons
Douglas	26	Cervical	5	Going to university
Ian	32	Thoracic	5	His new role as a parent

* The individuals' names have been changed to maintain confidentiality.

Interviews as data collection method

Data collection took the form of in-depth semi-structured interviews. At this point it is worth briefly discussing the topic of the research interview in more detail. Several approaches may be taken to interviews, depending on the choice of research design. The distinction is usually made between structured and unstructured interviews. According to Fontana and Frey (1994), structured interviewing refers to a situation in which an interviewer asks each respondent a series of pre-established questions with a limited set of response categories. The fixed order and number of questions resembles a script, which allows a degree of control over the interview. The structured interview is characteristic of quantitative or survey research, when the goal is to analyse the data statistically. This type of interviewing requires that the interviewer play a neutral role, establishing a casual rapport but without personal involvement. Unstructured interviewing derives from the ethnographic tradition in which the interviewer enters the interview with a list of issues to be covered, rather than deciding beforehand the exact questions they want to ask.

The ethnographic interview

Hammersley and Atkinson (1995) describe the ethnographic interview as semi-structured. These interviews are closer in character to complex conversations during which the interviewer may be a neutral listener or, on occasions, steer the direction taken by the interview as required to sustain the flow of the conversation. Non-directive questions are relatively open-ended and require a detailed answer rather than a specific piece of information or a simple 'yes' or 'no'. In non-directive interviewing the interviewer must be an active listener in order to assess how what is being said relates to the research focus and how it may reflect the circumstances of the interview (Hammersley & Atkinson 1995). Traditionally the aim has been to minimize the influence of the researcher on what the person says in response to the questions, although some directive or probing questions may be necessary in order for the interview to stay relatively on track. Staying on track also means that the researcher avoids getting involved in a real conversation, in which questions are asked of the interviewer by the participant, or personal opinions on the matters being discussed are solicited of the interviewer.

Fontana and Frey (1994) join feminist authors (see, for example, Reinharz 1992 and Smith 1987) in challenging these traditional qualitative interviewing techniques. The emphasis is shifting to allow the development of a closer relationship between the interviewer and the research participant, in an attempt to minimize status differences and do away with the traditional hierarchical situation in interviewing (Fontana & Frey 1994). This literature has resulted in an ongoing debate about the degree to which interviewers can engage more fully in the interview conversations, respond to questions, state opinions and react empathetically. Methodologically this new approach provides a greater spectrum of responses and a greater insight into respondents' or participants' perspectives (Reinharz 1992). The interview becomes part of a reciprocal interaction between the interviewer and the individual, who is describing their everyday reality. Preserving the viewpoint of the participants expresses a commitment to preserving the integrity of the phenomenon being investigated and comes closer to the phenomenological sensibility (Holstein & Gubrium 1994).

I have described the interviews I conducted for this study as semi-structured, for the following reasons: the questions were open-ended, broad and non-directive (Box 3.1), but were designed with the specific research goal in mind; and the data analysis involved direct transcription of the participants' verbal responses. An interview schedule consisting of a list of potential questions was developed from which a few could be selected during each interview, and there was no particular sequencing of the questions. Varying the questions accommodated for the individual styles of the people being interviewed.

On most occasions two or three questions were sufficient to produce a wealth of information and insights, but when necessary my professional experience did enable me to probe more deeply on specific topics and issues that the participant initiated as a result of a particular question. The in-depth responses to the questions clearly illustrated the reflective process that these individuals were engaged upon in relation to their disability and their lives.

Box 3.1 Examples of non-directive questions used in the interviews

◆ What would you describe about your experience to someone newly injured or to someone who knows nothing about spinal cord injury and its consequences?

◆ What would you describe as being 'successfully' rehabilitated? Would this describe you? What things have you done (or have others done) to assist you to reach this point in your life?

◆ Have your feelings about the experience of spinal cord injury changed in any way during the years since your injury?

◆ Before your injury, did you have any involvement or contact with a person with a disability resulting from spinal cord injury? If so, can you describe your reactions to that person?

◆ Has there ever been a time when your way of thinking about the experience of spinal cord injury seemed different from that of those people around you?

◆ Is there anyone you know who thinks about spinal cord injury and its consequences differently from you; for example, other individuals with the same injury, health professionals, friends or strangers?

◆ Imagine the years since your injury as a journey. Could you describe what has been most significant to you (influenced you the most) during that journey?

◆ How have you come to grips with what spinal cord injury and the resulting disability means to you and your life?

◆ How does this experience and the person you are today relate to the person you saw yourself as being before the injury?

◆ Is there anyone you know who is not making it through the experience of spinal cord injury, and do you know why not?

PILOT STUDY

Pilot studies are generally recommended, and prior to beginning this study I conducted interviews with two individuals who were interested in the study but who did not meet the exact criteria, as they had sustained a spinal cord injury over 10 years before. The results of these interviews strengthened my research design and data collection process in the following ways:

• The effectiveness of my interviewing technique was enhanced.
• Potential questions were tested.

• The reality of effective use of time was recognized.

• The unpredictability of the participants' verbal and emotional responses during the interview was illustrated, reinforcing the importance of being prepared to stop the interview and address the issues raised as a result of the questions.

• Explanation of the purpose of the research study was clarified as a result of feedback provided by these two individuals.

• During the course of the study participants informally acknowledged how important some of the issues raised during the interviews were to them, and expressed the wish that making them public would contribute to the education of rehabilitation professionals. Several of the participants read the published version of the study and affirmed its relevance both to their lives and to those providing rehabilitation services.

Some of the participants became almost angry when asked the open-ended, interpretive questions during the pilot study. They expressed this discomfort in questions, such as: 'Am I telling you what you want? What information do you need exactly? What are you trying to get at?'

All the participants knew of my connection with the rehabilitation centre, and it became obvious that they had made assumptions about the nature of the interview based on their experience of being interviewed by therapists in the rehabilitation setting, when questions are predictable and focused on acquiring specific information. Their confusion is indicative, and may be an indictment (depending on one's point of view) of the clinician-driven agenda informing clinical interviews and the conditioning of individuals to the patient role. It also became apparent, after reviewing the interview transcripts of the pilot study, that these individuals had redefined the direction of the interview and had assumed that my primary interest as a physical therapist was their rehabilitation in the institutional setting. It had not been my intention in this study to explore their experiences during hospitalization in either the acute care or the rehabilitation settings. As a result of the information gained from the pilot study I was able to revise the interview schedule, being careful to omit any reference to terms such as rehabilitation or treatment. In subsequent interviews I stressed my more general interest as a researcher in adult education.

The interviews were conducted at times and locations (home, office, a restaurant) chosen by the participants, and each lasted between $1\frac{1}{2}$ and 2 hours. All were audiotaped and transcribed, the transcripts forming the main data for the study.

ANALYSING DATA

Data analysis is a dynamic process weaving together recognition of emerging themes, identification of key ideas or units of meaning, and material acquired from the literature. The process often begins before all the interviews are completed. In this study each transcript was examined closely for phrases, sentences or paragraphs (i.e. participant quotes) which stood out as being meaningful and central to my broad area of research interest. These quotes were described as units of meaning, for example: 'I'd go somewhere else in my mind, go to a happy place. If they [the nurses] had a problem, it would snap me back to reality. Eventually, I began to realize that it was still my body and I had better attend to it a bit more' (Randy). This abstracting of data from the transcripts involved choices on my part, and constituted the first step of the interpretive process.

A systematic method of data organization described by Hammersley and Atkinson (1995) as 'physical sorting' was used in this study. This can be achieved in a variety of ways: by mounting data on large sheets of paper; by recording on file cards or in computer files; or by drawing a concept map (Clifford 1997). The units of meaning were physically assigned to a number of emerging themes or concepts, initially in file folders and later on large sheets of paper mounted on my living-room walls. This had the advantage of portraying the data

as a whole, as well as displaying the themes side by side for comparison.

Some of the themes arose spontaneously from the participants' interview responses, for example the use of jail terminology in their descriptions of their experiences in the rehabilitation centre. The interpretive process continued as the initial eight or nine themes were developed into three interconnected thematic categories (Carpenter 1994):

- rediscovering self
- redefining disability
- establishing a new identity.

The thematic categories are in this way grounded in the data, being both constructed by the researcher and abstracted from the language used by the participants. Detailed definitions were developed for each of these categories. The disadvantage of preconceived ideas which might flaw or limit the interpretive process was anticipated. A colleague, who possessed knowledge of spinal cord injury and qualitative research, was asked to identify units of meaning from intact transcript copies and to assign them to the categories using the definitions established. Discrepancies which arose between our respective decisions caused me to reflect and to more clearly define the categories. The data analysis process I experienced was circular in nature, rather than sequential. Each transcript brought new information and insights, and caused me to re-evaluate the emerging themes and my definitions of the final three thematic categories, and this sent me back to the literature.

FINDINGS

The scope of this chapter allows only a brief description of the actual findings (for more details see Carpenter 1994). The three categories of description identified in this study – rediscovering self, redefining disability and establishing a new identity – by which meaning was made of the injury, represented commonalities but also revealed the complex and multidimensional nature of each individual's experience.

Rediscovering self

The injury and overall sense of loss experienced, particularly in the early post-injury stages, were symbolized for the participants by the physical changes resulting from the injury or the external experience of disability. These were seen as being separate from the internal concept of self, which was perceived as being the same as pre-injury and which represented their accumulated life history and experience. The category of rediscovering self was described as being concerned with resolving the split between the internal and external selves. This split was evident in the paradoxical nature of some of the participants' comments, for example: 'I've definitely changed since my injury. I'm pretty much the same person I was before' (David).

The rehabilitation programme was seen as contributing to this experiential split by its emphasis on the negative physical ramifications of the injury. Although the participants acknowledged that the programme provided important information about altered physiological functioning and the skills essential for survival following the injury, it was also experienced as a restrictive and isolating environment: 'You've got to get your two years in, it's like doing hard time, like being in jail' (Brian). Dirk, trying to explain how rehabilitation contributed to a sense of separation from his real world, said: 'On discharge it was difficult to cope and get back into a family lifestyle. You have to relearn how to live with people again.' Whereas the participants appreciated the support and assistance provided by individual professionals, they also recognized, with hindsight, how influenced they were by the emphasis on the limiting consequences of the injury, and expressed frustration at the invocation of expected accomplishments related to level of injury: for example, Brian commented that: 'People told me things at first which kinda blew me away, like the physical therapist who just baldly told me "you can't do that at your level".'

The process of regaining a coherent sense of self was found to be facilitated by acknowledging self-responsibility, for example:

'It's my life', the development of a new framework of disability experience, and the passage of time. Returning to the real world represented a new series of disturbing insights related to accepting self-responsibility, for example: 'I had to accept that I'm more vulnerable' (William), and 'Ultimately it's you who has to come out of it. I mean everyone can tell you what to do and what's good for you but in the end it's you who has to become the expert' (Randy). There is a sense of things falling into place, of life going on fairly normally, and of getting back on track as the experiential split is narrowed and a sense of the old self is rediscovered. Learning, which to this point has been primarily related to skill acquisition, begins to assume a more reflective quality. As Larry said: 'Far away from the hospital experience I can evaluate what I've assimilated and what I've learned and I'll tell you I'm impressed with the changes.'

Redefining disability

The category of redefining disability describes the efforts and strategies used by individuals to change their own subjective experience of disability. Central to redefining disability was the need to challenge the stereotypes and attitudes associated with disability which the participants experienced as being held by many health professionals, and which were seen to influence the way in which they interacted with their patients. The gradual rediscovery of self appeared to provide the participants with an avenue by which a personal interpretation of disability could be made, in terms not of inadequacy or limitations, but of personal potential, expertise and self-confidence. Redefining disability involved challenging the expectations of health professionals and regaining a sense of personal coherence (for example, 'I'm back on track'), and enabled the individuals to carve out their own definitions of 'normal' and 'disability'. In asserting their own vision of life with a disability – albeit initially a shaky vision – these individuals spoke of slowly gaining confidence in their own capabilities as 'the expert', and beginning to trust their interpretations of new situations. The reality of living with a disability in society was consistently referred to by the subjects as an adventure. They identified themselves as being the sort of people who would 'just get out there and do it', and in their opinion it was this characteristic that contributed most to their perceived success post injury. The disability, instead of being experienced as a personal trait, appeared to have become a set of physical characteristics that influenced function. The participants' accounts emphasized the element of personal growth inherent in redefining disability, as well as their conviction of the fundamental importance of non-physical values, such as relationships with others, kindness, cooperation, doing one's best, and patience. As Dirk said: 'All the things I thought were really important before I now find were not. Like at first what bothered me was that I wouldn't be able to throw a ball to my sons any more. You think at first that you've lost more than you have. We're much closer in a different way now. Where you come from is the heart, and I think just that insight is a gain.'

Establishing a new identity

Establishing a new identity is described as being concerned with the roles that identify and describe the individual as a social being, and which are central to a person's self-concept. The roles identified by the participants were spouse or lover, parent, employee, sports team member, student, and church participant. These roles contributed to a generalized vision of themselves as individuals. This vision is an amalgam of abilities, talents, defects and overall independent functioning by which the self is revealed to others. It is consequently closely related to body image. Immediately following spinal cord injury a whole series of 'I ams', mentioned by the participants in the past tense, such as 'I was tall', 'I was an athlete' or 'I was a fisherman', are no longer relevant and a loss of identity is experienced. The learning process revealed by the participants involved

letting go of some 'I ams' and developing others about which they could feel good. Ian, prior to his injury, had not given much thought to having children, but post injury he felt 'as if my daughter is the result of all the changes I've gone through, that I'm a much better father than I would have been, and that's so positive'.

This process was found to be associated with making comparisons with others by which self-esteem could be enhanced; by association and dialogue with a peer minority ('the brothers in arms'); by creating intimacy with significant others and new ways of interacting with society; and by becoming 'managers of social interactions'.

In summary, the continuity of self was of primary importance to the ongoing experience of disability, and the learning strategies involved were diverse and intensely personal. The key, it seems, is perceiving disability as a part of the picture of the continuum of a person's life, not as pervading the whole (Carpenter 1994).

THE RESEARCHER ROLE

Central to this type of research is the concept of reflexivity which, according to Hammersley and Atkinson (1995), 'implies that the orientations of the researcher will be shaped by their socio-historical locations, including the values and interests that these locations confer' (p. 16). The concept of reflexivity suggests that striving to eliminate the effects of the researcher is futile; rather, the role of the researcher needs to be thoroughly monitored and discussed. Such information enables the reader to interact critically with the study. This interactive process includes gaining insights about the phenomenon being studied, an understanding of the perspective of the participants and their interaction with the researcher, questioning problematic components and seeking further information.

It is generally agreed that in qualitative research the researcher is the key instrument (see Chapter 10), and that their understanding, theoretical knowledge and insights are brought to bear on all aspects of the research process. It was important for me, in this study, to meticulously monitor and document my impact as researcher. A number of strategies were used to achieve this goal, and these can be grouped under the following headings:

- The researcher's authenticity
- Relationship with the participants
- Establishment of trust and rapport
- Data organization and analysis
- Reflective strategies used
- Impact on personal view of the phenomenon being studied.

The researcher's authenticity

My experience as a clinician, my familiarity with the consequences of spinal cord injury, and my theoretical background in rehabilitation and adult education grounded the research and directed the research process, and represented my claim to authenticity as a researcher. It is important in qualitative research that the researcher's position be clearly documented (see Chapter 10). It is this documentation that supports the reflexive nature of the research. As a result of my experience and knowledge I was familiar with the terminology related to spinal cord injury and its consequences used by the participants, was able to respond quickly to issues arising in the interviews, and was able to be both an active listener and a participant in the interview process.

Relationship with participants

All the individuals involved in the study were aware of my professional interest in and knowledge of spinal cord injury, and several already knew me from the rehabilitation centre. Although far from being an 'insider' to the experiences of spinal cord injury, my understanding and knowledge of the day-to-day realities of the resulting disability meant that the participants did not feel they had to explain references to the physical consequences of the injury, for example problems with bladder and

bowel functioning or spasticity. This meant that the responses to the questions assumed a broader and more reflective quality. In this way, my professional expertise and accumulated knowledge of spinal cord injury could be seen as valuable tools in the data collection process.

Some of the issues raised during the interviews were of an intimate and emotional nature, and I was keenly aware that I had a responsibility to provide the names of resources who would be able to address any issues that remained unresolved for the individual at the end of the interview. This was not in fact necessary, but I did feel the need to consider the possible impact of my research on those who had volunteered to share their experiences with me.

Establishment of trust and rapport

The interviews were conducted at a location of the participant's choosing, and were frequently preceded by general conversation and, occasionally, cups of tea. In this way a relaxed atmosphere was created and rapport established. I made it clear that at any time, if the individual wished, the tape would be stopped. This occurred on two occasions and an in-depth conversation ensued that was not considered part of the research project. The interview was continued only at the individual's request. In this way I tried to establish my own integrity and ensure that, if required, the participants could assume a measure of control over the process. Gaining trust is enhanced by the researcher showing genuine feelings and responding honestly to comments and questions posed by the participants; it is an integral element of qualitative research.

Data analysis

As the researcher, I was intimately involved with every phase of the research process. The idea of researcher as instrument is a central characteristic of qualitative research. My clinical experience, observations and knowledge, and my exploration of the literature constituted my subjectivity as a researcher and definitely influenced the data analysis and interpretation. As Bailey (1997) points out, qualitative research *is* by definition subjective: it is this subjectivity that contributes to the richness and depth of the data. A number of strategies relating to researcher 'bias' and which can be used to enhance the trustworthiness of the research are discussed in Chapter 10. Every effort has to be made to ensure that the emerging themes or categories are thoroughly grounded in the data; this entails many rereadings of the transcripts and revisions of category definitions. Throughout the data analysis the emphasis must be on presenting an accurate portrayal of the participant's reality. The imperative is to make transparent the reflexive process by which the study findings were obtained.

Reflective strategies

I used two strategies to supplement the data and facilitate my own reflective process: notes made as I re-listened to the taped interviews, and 'analytic memos' (Hammersley & Atkinson 1995). The notes I made directly on to the transcripts enabled me to capture the details that were unique to each interview; for example, how I felt about the way I asked probing questions, and thoughts on the meaning of what a participant was really saying during an exchange that seemed important. Throughout the process of interviewing and reading transcripts and related literature, I experienced, in an ongoing fashion, new theoretical insights which were recorded in the form of analytic memos. An example of such a memo was:

I've just realized the language being used to describe the wheelchair function is different – phrases like 'good balance', 'turns well', 'light', and 'looks cool' – from that I associate with wheelchair use. 'Being in' a wheelchair usually reflects stigma. Contrast this positive use with how the media and health professionals think of wheelchair use – 'in', 'confined to', and 'restricted to' a wheelchair. Transformation of wheelchair as symbol of disability to one of mobility and capability.

The compilation of such memos represents the sort of 'internal dialogue or thinking aloud' (Hammersley & Atkinson 1995) that is the essence of the reflexive nature of qualitative research. These memos enabled me to trace the way my intellectual process was shaping the preliminary data analysis.

Impact on personal view of the phenomenon being studied

The experience of conducting this study made a significant impact on my view of disability as part of the continuum of an adult's life, and provided some largely unexpected insights into the individual's perspective of rehabilitation practice.

My physical therapy education had been based on the restoration of optimal *physical* function, and I came to realize how closely I associated this function with quality of life. This narrow definition of quality of life was clearly refuted by the participants' diverse descriptions of their experience of spinal cord injury.

I also recognized, for the first time in a long career in rehabilitation, how dominant psychological and sociological theories, in particular stages of adjustment and normalization theories, and what Oliver (1990, p. 10) has called the 'personal tragedy view of disability', had influenced my practice and attitude towards disability (for a brief overview of these theories see Hammell 1992). As a result of my in-depth interactions with individuals with spinal cord injury and the qualitative research process, I was challenged to reflect on my own interpretation of disability and my attitudes towards the value systems of clients in rehabilitation that give rise to their personal goals and aspirations. This study clearly illustrated the need for rehabilitation professionals to revisit the concept of successful rehabilitation, not in terms of skills acquisition, but in terms of what is relevant and important to individuals in the context of their own lives.

REFERENCES

Bailey DM 1997 Research for the health professional: a practical guide, 2nd edn. FA Davis, Philadelphia

Carpenter C 1994 The experience of spinal cord injury: the individual's perspective – implications for rehabilitation practice. Physical Therapy 74(7):614–629

Clifford C 1997 Qualitative research methodology. Churchill Livingstone, New York

Dohrenwend BS, Dohrenwend BP (eds) 1974 Stressful life events: their nature and effects. John Wiley & Sons, New York

Fontana A, Frey JH 1994 Interviewing: the art of science. In: Denzin NK, Lincoln YS (eds) Handbook of qualitative research. Sage Publishing, London, pp 361–376

Hammell KW 1992 Psychological and sociological theories concerning adjustment to traumatic spinal cord injury: the implications for rehabilitation. Paraplegia 30:317–326

Hammersley M, Atkinson P 1995 Ethnography: principles in practice, 2nd edn. Routledge, London

Holstein JA, Gubrium JF 1994 Phenomenology, ethnomethodology, and interpretive practice. In: Denzin NK, Lincoln YS (eds) Handbook of qualitative research. Sage Publishing, London, pp 262–272

Oliver M 1990 The politics of disablement. Macmillan, Basingstoke

Reinharz S 1992 Feminist methods in social research. Oxford University Press, Oxford, pp 18–45

Smith D 1987 The everyday world as problematic: a feminist sociology. Northeastern University Press, Boston

FURTHER READING

Carpenter C 1997 Conducting qualitative research in physiotherapy. Physiotherapy 83(10):547–552

Denzin NK, Lincoln YS (eds) 1994 Introduction: Entering the field of qualitative research. In: Handbook of Qualitative Research. Sage Publishing, London, pp 1–17

Domholdt E 1993 Research paradigms. In: Physical therapy research: principles and applications. WB Saunders, Philadelphia, pp 121–140

Miles MB, Huberman AM 1994 Qualitative data analysis: an expanded sourcebook. Sage, Thousand Oaks, CA

Shepard KF, Gwyer J, Hack LM, Jensen GM, Schmoll BJ 1993 Alternative approaches to research in physical therapy: positivism and phenomenology. Physical Therapy 73(2):88–97

4

Issues related to data collection

Melinda Suto

OVERVIEW

Data collection sounds like a straightforward aspect of qualitative research. Methods are learned, incorporated into the research design, and evaluated for their efficacy. The reality of designing and conducting projects becomes more complex when the participants involved constitute a particularly vulnerable population. In this case the researcher is required to weigh the advantages and disadvantages of various strategies against emergent ethical issues. To illuminate some of the problems encountered and the strategies used in such studies, this chapter draws on research about how people with chronic schizophrenia use time and the environment to enact their daily occupations. The objectives of this chapter are to:

- analyse the use of selected data collection strategies with an emphasis on participant observation and ethnographic interviews
- discuss the triangulation of data collection methods
- explore such ethical issues as informed consent and power relations that challenge researchers who attempt to understand something about the lives of marginalized individuals.

The choice of interviewing and participant observation has the potential to uncover the power differential between health-care researchers and the people with mental illnesses who allow us into their lives. Any insights gained through the research process must be shared with other therapists to enable them to engage in therapy that begins from the client's viewpoint. The aim of this chapter is to eventually benefit the lives of people whose very symptoms and behaviours at best elicit misunderstanding, and at worst fail to arouse interest from the research community.

TEMPORAL PERSPECTIVE IN THE ROLES AND OCCUPATIONS OF PEOPLE WITH CHRONIC SCHIZOPHRENIA

Occupational therapists whose research questions emerge from foreshadowed problems or the puzzlements of their practice often bring a passion to research that sustains their interest and enables them to complete the project. My interest lies in determining how occupational therapists can understand the complex relationship between time, the environment and the individual with chronic schizophrenia, and use that knowledge to change the services offered to this population. Ten years of observing the difficulties that people with chronic schizophrenia have in structuring their time to enable meaningful occupations for themselves prompted an extensive literature review. The literature confirmed my anecdotal experience, but revealed little about the association between temporal perspective and the individual's ability to orchestrate and enact daily occupations to fulfil socially and culturally expected roles. 'Temporal perspective' refers to the understanding of past events and expectations of the future. The research thus focuses on the following questions:

• What daily, weekly, monthly and yearly activities structure life for people with chronic schizophrenia who live in a board and care home? (Board and care home is a term used in Canada and the United States that usually refers to large residential facilities with little or no provision for rehabilitation or other services. A

similar facility in Britain falls under the domain of sheltered housing, and in Australia it is called supported accommodation.)
• How is future time perspective demonstrated in the actions and talk of these individuals?
• Is there any relationship between the quantity and quality of self-initiated goal-directed actions demonstrated and the individual's future time perspective?

A brief overview of the research design, subject selection and findings is presented as a framework for the larger discussion of data collection experiences and ethical issues. For a full description of the research see Suto and Frank (1994).

RESEARCH DESIGN

The nature of the questions posed helps determine the choice of research methodology. Working within a qualitative paradigm allows observation, description and analysis of daily occupations within the context in which they naturally occur. The qualitative methods I chose included participant observation, ethnographic interviews, access to public and personal documents and self-reported time-use logs. I observed 10 selected residents within a board and care home and surrounding community for 9 weeks, and recorded 76 hours of participant observation in the form of field notes. These notes detailed conversations, activities and observations about the participants, the staff and the environment (Emerson et al 1995). Field notes formed the primary recorded data of these interactions, and also included my impressions, questions and concerns about the process and my role as researcher. The personal documents accessed were confined to the health-care/facility record of each participant, and the limited information obtained was incorporated into the field notes. Conversely, information about the residential facility was readily available. The field notes were analysed thematically both during the data collection period and after the on-site interactions ceased. Semi-structured interviews were conducted with nine of the 10 participants in the middle 3 weeks of the period of participant observation. The semi-structured interviews and self-reported time-use logs were used to *triangulate* the data (see Chapter 10). The self-reported time-use logs were not consistently completed by the participants, and in reality the information was only of minimal help in triangulating the data and will therefore not be discussed in any great detail.

Participant selection is an integral part of the research design. A group of 50 people resided in this licensed facility situated in a large American city. Ten individuals who met the DSM-III-R criteria for chronic schizophrenia participated in the research (American Psychiatric Association 1987). The ages of the five women and five men ranged from 29 to 60 years. Staff suggested several individuals as potential participants because of their high functioning status. This subjective judgement was based on money management, transportation, social interaction and other skills that differentiated these residents from their peers. Three of the participants identified themselves as African-American when asked to describe their ethnic or cultural identity, and the remaining seven gave 'white' as their response.

RESEARCH FINDINGS

The research findings demonstrate that formal or institutional structures are used by the facility to orient residents to the present and immediate future. This future is proximal rather than distal: it typically refers to later the same day. Formal structures are identified from routines (daily, weekly, and other times) within the environment that include scheduled mealtimes, medication allocation and money distribution. These proximal temporal markers give predictability to the residents' days and reference points that may guide their actions and increase their general awareness of time. They do not, however, encourage the development of future time perspective in residents for their own plans. The formal structures seem inadvertently to impede the development of personal habits that might support greater independence in daily occupations. Informal or phenomenological structures are created by routines and activities initiated by residents, staff members or a combination of both. In contrast to the formal facility structures, these occurrences are predicated on the residents' personal habits, the desired pace (timing) of activities, and the availability of resources.

That having a future time perspective enhances the likelihood of self-initiated goal-directed behaviour was supported by the data. Participants who made plans beyond the day also engaged in a greater number of observable goal-directed activities than their peers. The comparison is grounded in empirical data that describe many residents who express no specific plans or whose plans are in the present. The quality of planned actions is determined in part by the feasibility of one's plans. Also, opportunities for goal-directed actions that support social roles in the facility are limited by its structure, the symptoms of chronic schizophrenia that many residents experience, and other contextual features. Thus activities that constitute roles, such as that of family member, hobbyist or paid worker, are severely limited. For example, the expectations of a family member might include visiting others, celebrating birthdays and other special events, and contributing financial or emotional support to family members. Limited finances to enable travel or long-distance telephone calls, and interpersonal difficulties associated with schizophrenia, can make such role functioning a challenge. These research findings reinforce the role of the environment as a critical mediator between the individual and the occupation in which they wish to engage. It allows an emphasis on people's plans and actions, rather than their symptoms.

CRITIQUE OF DATA COLLECTION STRATEGIES

Participant observation

Anthropology and sociology practices provide historical precedence for the use of participant observation and, along with other social science disciplines. continue to critique and refine this research strategy (Atkinson & Hammersley 1994). Participant observation is both a role the researcher plays and a method for collecting data within the context of people's lives. In this study it involved socializing with residents in common areas, sharing meals, accompanying people on errands in the community, and talking with staff. The approach requires non-judgemental listening, but also focused questioning. The aim is to blend somewhat into the milieu and, through participation, obtain a better understanding of events and conversations than is possible by observation alone. Participant observation requires ongoing negotiations and decisions about what, when, where and how to involve oneself. Although the need for gathering any data seems to prevail initially, conducting data analysis throughout the project can guide the researcher's decisions.

After gaining approval for the research project from the owners and the residents of the board and care facility, I began 9 weeks of participant observation. Communicating my role to the residents and staff involved introducing myself as a graduate student in occupational therapy and explaining the project. I gave some residents a brief description of my role; others heard the detailed explanation based on their interest or my wish to include them as research participants. The emphasis on student versus therapist was deliberate and reinforced by my questions and non-authoritative manner. For example, I attended a crafts activity which ended with participants receiving tickets (chits) that I assumed were probably redeemable for privileges, food treats or something extra. In order to check this assumption, I asked different residents to explain how chits are used and what they think about the system.

Recording the data from participant observation sessions accurately is accomplished by writing field notes immediately after each visit and before discussing the experiences with anyone else. Field notes that are developed after talking about the session risk losing the fresh descriptive nature in favour of generalization or

analysis. The intrusive nature of audio or videotaping, as well as the ethical problem of including people who have not signed consent forms, requires the researcher to develop a good memory and jot down key words and phrases inconspicuously. I would leave the room periodically to write notes in an office, washroom or other area away from the residents. My departures fitted into an environment where people moved about frequently and seemingly drew little notice from others. As each hour in the field requires 2–3 hours of narrative-style writing, participant observation sessions of 1–2 hours produced the most accurate, concrete renditions of behaviours, conversations and subjective impressions.

Coding the data occurs by reading the field notes, identifying emerging themes and then categorizing relevant chunks of data. Ongoing data coding is essential for cueing the researcher to pursue different themes and realize when thematic categories are saturated. For example, data collected for the category I termed 'activities structured by staff' became repetitive about halfway through the project. This realization directed my thinking about how residents create routines and initiate goal-directed actions. Ongoing data analysis indicated that some thematic categories became saturated earlier than others. For example, I realized that data categorized under 'responses to the researcher' soon became repetitious. The recognition that no substantially new responses to my presence seemed forthcoming allowed me to limit collection of those kinds of data and focus on interpersonal communication instead.

Participant observation was appropriately selected to address the kinds of research questions outlined earlier. Despite the undisputed usefulness of this method, four issues remain that warrant consideration, with the hope that future studies may benefit from this discussion. First, managing to shed my occupational therapy role, with its attendant behaviours, expectations and world view, was not easy. Although prior experience of working in mental health settings helped me remain non-directive, the urge to intervene when a solution appeared obvious and simply obtained was tempting. For example, in the arts and crafts group there were opportunities to assist people and allow them to proceed to the next step more quickly. Most of the time I resisted the desire to facilitate in such group settings because it might have altered the milieu I was trying to understand. Given the long hours of unstructured time available to residents, I had many different ideas for groups and restructuring the environment. I usually negotiated this urge to intervene by asking open-ended questions and giving opinions occasionally. This approach reinforced my role as a learner in the setting. Most residents identified social services as quite beneficial to them. Therefore, it was not too difficult to contain my professional actions in conversations and interviews. The ability to blend into the environment is made easier by dressing casually, 'hanging out', smoking, and drinking coffee or soft drinks. Monitoring any overwhelming extroverted behaviours is advisable. For example, a loquacious, bubbly presentation and other distracting personality features that might disrupt the milieu and affect the kinds of data collected should be avoided.

The second challenge of being a participant observer is to remain non-judgemental and appear to be interested in people's stories. The repetition of stories can be tiring to hear, frustrating in their inconsistency, and occasionally boring. It is difficult to judge whether on this occasion the individual's comments might yield useful insights to further the research goals. Towards the end of one's time in the field especially, feelings of boredom may signal the need to change focus, or indicate that a category is sufficiently saturated with data.

A third issue that may arise during participant observation is the researcher's awareness that rules or laws are being broken. The negotiation of ethical or legal dilemmas is influenced partly by the researcher's values and partly by the severity of the offence. The consequences of 'whistle-blowing' on the researcher's subsequent credibility and ability to continue gathering data are also a consideration.

I was aware of several instances of residents drinking liquor in their rooms and smoking marijuana. Smoking illegal drugs is a civil offence and both actions breach stated facility rules. Although there may be adverse consequences to taking psychotropic medication with alcohol and street drugs, I did not judge the residents to be at sufficient risk to warrant disclosure to the facility staff. If the drug deals and assaults so common to the community in which the board and care facility was situated had involved residents, my action would have been quite different.

Time is the final issue to consider when selecting participant observation. This refers to the actual chunks of time over a period of weeks or months, and the time necessary to write field notes from those sessions. The 76 hours of onsite data collection over 9 weeks allowed me to complete the research goals. However, I question what insights were missed by not interacting with residents for a full cycle, such as an entire year. Would I have made different conclusions about the effect of the environment on the participants' goal-directed behaviours? Participant observation is often limited by practical constraints, i.e. how much release time is available from one's other work responsibilities. In summary, issues of role negotiation, interpersonal behaviours, broken rules and temporal constraints require careful attention when engaging in participant observation. The next section discusses the relevance of these issues as part of the critique of using ethnographic interviews.

Ethnographic interviews

One of the guiding principles behind ethnographic interviewing is an openness to the participant's point of view (Bogdan & Biklen 1998, Fontana & Frey 1994). The use of open-ended questions within a semi-structured interview format helps the researcher appreciate the participant's perspective. This style of interaction encourages the narrative to unfold according to the participant's direction and personal storytelling style. It facilitates the production of highly descriptive data and offers opportunities for the researcher to ask probing questions periodically, thereby focusing their learning. I conducted interviews with nine of the 10 participants in the middle 3 weeks of the participant observation period. The rapport I developed with them and the acquisition of signed consent forms influenced when the interviews were scheduled.

In contrast to the participant observer role, being an interviewer required less role negotiation. It was not difficult to maintain interest in participants' stories. Each interview was an efficient way to collect data with few distractions. Interviews began with closed-type questions to create a demographic database for the study and ease the participant into the questioning process. I had control over the interview in the sense of being able to ask various questions. The participants held ultimate control, however, and could determine the extent and veracity of the information they provided. For example, Jeff, one of the residents who was given several work responsibilities by staff, raised the issue of some residents drinking alcohol. This arose in the context of a discussion about loaning money. The unsolicited information furthered my knowledge about house rules and their exemptions, systems of money management, and reasons for interpersonal connections between residents. The description of drinking confirmed my impression of Jeff as a key informant within the setting. That status was based on observing the tasks he completed and listening to what staff and other residents said about his level of responsibility at the home.

The interviews furthered the goals of research but caused obvious anxiety for some participants. Anxiety may have prompted two participants to refuse the option of having the interviews audiotaped. Alternatively, this choice may have stemmed from other reasons related to their condition, such as paranoia. The refusal is significant because it challenges the power differential between the participant and the researcher. I felt ambivalence about the authority and power granted to me as a researcher, although without some authority I might have

been unsuccessful in obtaining cooperation from the participants. With the benefit of hindsight, I view each instance of someone refusing to participate in the research, to complete a 24-hour time log, or just to chat with me, as a potentially assertive and healthy response. The power differential highlighted by an interview structure in which the researcher asks the questions is particularly relevant when working with individuals who have mental illness. Talk alone cannot change the balance of social power or perceived status, but sincere appreciation of the participant's time and willingness to talk is helpful. A statement that the participant can refuse to answer some questions, when supported by action, shows respect for the individual. A variation of this practice occurred when half of the participants refused to complete 24-hour activity time logs that I distributed after 5 weeks in the field. A more persistent researcher might have obtained a greater number of completed time logs. Acceptance of those refusals can be criticized, but such are the consequences of negotiating my role rather than trying to impose my will. The difficulty with completing the time logs with the level of detail that would have been useful was not anticipated prior to selecting the method. The use of time logs did not constitute a strong data collection method, despite providing some support for activity patterns I had already observed or heard about.

Public and personal documents

Documents can be a rich source of information that may be challenged or confirmed by data collected through participant observation and interview. The main public documents available in the board and care home were brochures describing the facility, schedules of special events and activities, facility routines, a poster outlining patients' rights, and various announcements posted on the corkboard. The monthly 'Regularly Scheduled Activities' notice listed enough pastimes to keep an energetic Club Med member busy! Gardening, music appreciation, nature walks, croquet, in-house library and exercises may indeed have occurred during the year, but did not appear to occur frequently. What often happened, according to a written schedule, were 'monthly residents' meetings; bingo; assistance with bath, shaving and medication, and arts and crafts' (Suto 1988). The entire posting left the mistaken impression of an environment with numerous daily activities from which to choose. These kinds of public documents formed the basis of information for prospective residents and interested professionals.

Personal documents from which data may be collected include, but are not limited to, diaries, letters, autobiographies, photographs, résumés and essays in either written form or some other media (Bogdan & Biklen 1998). The resident's chart was the primary personal document accessible to me. The relatively brief time in the field precluded the development of any close relationships with participants in which more personal documents might be shared.

The administrator appropriately denied me access to any resident's chart until I had presented signed consent forms for each file. This situation necessitated reliance on the administrator's judgement to identify potential participants to me, based on the selection criteria for the research project. His assistance with suggesting which residents might be interested and how to find them was essential, given the limited time available to complete the research.

The facility documents on each participant confirmed the research inclusion criteria, e.g. diagnosis, age, and absence of organic brain pathology. Some demographic and historical data were also available. In some instances many years of health-care history were condensed to hospital admission dates recorded on a one-page 'face' sheet. Frequently information was incomplete, even for residents who had lived at the facility for many years. Neither the demographic data nor the past health-care history was particularly useful in meeting the research goals. In other settings, however, broadly defined personal and public documents may prove effective in furthering the research goals. The next section offers a closer

examination of triangulation, an incorporation of different data collection methods and sources into the research design.

TRIANGULATION OF DATA

Data methods

The use of multiple data collection strategies forms part of the triangulation process and strengthens the credibility of the research finding (Krefting 1991, Janesick 1994). Three data collection methods, critiqued earlier as separate entities, are now reviewed together, drawing upon examples from the same research project. The large number of people in the board and care home and management's attitude allowed me to amass participant observation data at any time. Although only 10 individuals consented to participate directly in the study, it was agreed that observations of the environment that excluded the other 40 residents would be misleading. It was beneficial to see what people do, rather than rely solely on self-report or other informants. Even my limited participation in the residents' daily activities changed my understanding of the relationship between the environment and their use of time.

The qualities of patience, unobtrusiveness, curiosity and discipline are necessary for successful participant observation. Despite my embodiment of these qualities, at times it was useful to gain an individual's complete attention and focus questions on a particular topic. In private interviews with the participants I used knowledge from observations and concepts from the literature to pose questions about time use. Questions that would seem out of context and intrusive in the 'living room' milieu were easily posed during interviews. The probes and requests for more detail were smoothly made between typical interview questions, such as: 'Could you describe an average weekday here?' and 'Do you have any plans or goals (things you want to do) in the next day? Week? Month?' Ten opinions were added to my own observations about the influence of scheduled activities on people's daily plans and strengthened the analysis of these data. Interviews also allowed me to make contact with participants who were taciturn or who rarely spent time in the common areas that I frequented.

Conducting individual interviews challenges the researcher's developing impressions about participants, the environment and the occupations within it. For example, the interview with Rosemary was fraught with inaccuracies in her personal history (compared to her chart) and instances of unusual thought patterns, yet Rosemary maintained a system of running errands for cash, making small loans that she remembered, and purchasing items from saved chits. The contrast between her observed occupational performance and the content and tangential nature of the interview prompted a revised perspective of Rosemary. This insight directed my focus to how the environment supported Rosemary's occupational function, perhaps even compensating for what appeared to be cognitive dysfunction.

Without interviews, I would have been limited to asking staff or other residents directly about a participant's behaviours, thoughts and feelings. Although comments on others' behaviour were appropriate and useful most of the time, feelings and thoughts are best obtained from each participant directly. Also, polling people would have contradicted the unobtrusive stance I tried to maintain. It was appropriate, however, to ask direct questions of staff and residents about how the board and care home was managed. Questions involved staffing, routines, conflict resolution, financial arrangements, and treatment approaches for residents, to name a few topics. It strengthened the research findings to obtain information from both groups of constituents about issues because of their predictably different perspectives. Two staff members in particular served as key informants who frequently responded at length to my questions and often provided unsolicited information. Multiple means of data collection encourages the cross-checking of facts and subjective comments, which increases the likelihood that one's findings represent the research setting and participants faithfully.

Ethnographic interviews alone would not have captured the complex social interactions that some of the seemingly less functional residents in particular managed. In a subsequent research project my questions focused on the understanding of leisure time and how it was used. I was interested in understanding what enables and impedes participation for individuals who have chronic mental health problems but who live outside hospitals or board and care facilities. Because of time constraints and the heterogeneity of the residential environments, ethnographic interviewing was the sole data collection method for this second project. This limitation resulted in a final product that was less satisfying than the first qualitative research study. An analysis of the interviews did produce an understanding of the problems and potential solutions regarding leisure. I would have had greater confidence in the findings, however, had I employed multiple data collection methods such as those described here. Triangulation through the use of different data methods and data sources is commonly practised, as the following section demonstrates. Researchers may also incorporate triangulation strategies such as diverse theoretical perspectives, multiple investigators and interdisciplinary viewpoints into their research designs (Janesick 1994).

Data sources

The diversity of '… time, space, and person in observation and interviewing' (Krefting 1991, p. 219) provided by the triangulation of data collection sources adds greatly to confidence in the research findings. Conducting participant observation at various times of the day, and on different days of the week, is important for several reasons. Different facility routines occur during evenings and weekends, and also the staff changes, which provides opportunities for new data collection. Board and care residents are offered options at weekends, such as popcorn and videos on Saturdays and ice cream on Sunday afternoons. Overall, there are fewer structured activities and of course no appointments to attend on weekends. The societal imperative of weekends is not lost on some of the residents: some use these times to visit family, go on recreational outings, attend church, and otherwise change their customary round of daily activities. Varying the time of day when participant observation occurs gives the researcher a more accurate impression of the milieu than attending only in the daytime, for example. Concerns for my personal safety in the neighbourhood influenced the times of participant observation considerably. Thus only 7 hours of participant observation occurred after 5:30 pm. Although unanticipated in the design of the research, this limitation constitutes a criticism of how the methods were employed.

Obtaining information from a variety of informants is preferable to relying on one group of people, regardless of the group's credibility. Many residents and various staff members expressed different opinions about the same issues and occurrences. These discrepancies arose in part from differences in roles, education levels, mental health status, and attitudes and knowledge about chronic mental illnesses. For example, here is the part-time cook's attitude to the residents: 'Well, I just put myself in their shoes. Everyone wants to be treated right' (Suto 1988). In contrast, one of the more 'educated' and generally compassionate co-owners stated: 'They're like children here; at least you have to treat them that way. You must always listen and be patient' (Suto 1988). There were also some differences of opinion between senior staff (owners and the assistant manager) and some residents about the range of activity options. Although it is necessary to consider the influence of schizophrenic symptoms on such comments, numerous residents mentioned the lack of activities available. Comments such as: 'I like to sleep a lot because there's nothing to do here anyway' contrast with staff perceptions and postings in the facility hallway (Suto 1988).

Participant observation lends itself to using diverse settings and groupings of people as data collection sources. Within the board and care home, private (offices and bedrooms) and more public areas (living room and kitchen) were the main venues for data collection. I was unable to participate in the few group outings offered, but did accompany several participants on short trips to the local stores. These opportunities allowed me to compare the participants' interactions with individuals other than staff, residents, visitors to the facility, and myself. Group configurations during participant observation ranged from small groups of four to nine women and men, to sessions in the living room with 10–30 people. The smaller groups were prevalent in structured settings, such as the weekly health lectures and the arts and crafts sessions. Interviews were always done privately and usually away from likely interruptions.

Lastly, seasons of the year and the duration of the researcher's time in the field offer options for data sources. Seasonal changes provide a glimpse of how holidays are celebrated by various participants in the setting. For example, who organizes Christmas festivities? Are other religious holidays such as Hanukkah also celebrated? Who decides what justifies a celebration? At the board and care home, weekend staff organized food and decorations for a 4th July (American) Independence Day party. Changes in the season in some environments necessitate increased amounts of time spent either indoors or outdoors. Given the unchanging temperate climate of the city in which the research occurred, it was unlikely that the lack of participant observation during other seasons affected the project findings. In an earlier discussion about participant observation issues, I identified the duration of the data collection period as potentially affecting the depth of information gathered. There are no set guidelines about how many weeks, for example, data collection should continue. The research questions, the settings, the number of participants and the available hours per day are all factors in determining what is an appropriate duration for data collection.

ETHICAL ISSUES OF STUDYING A VULNERABLE POPULATION

The ethical issues that arise when contemplating and conducting research with a vulnerable population of marginalized people differ from those relevant to some other groups. Proposed research projects have long been subject to approval by the ethical review boards of hospitals, universities and other public and private 'gatekeepers'. In addition, in the years since the completion of this board and care home research, advocacy groups representing people with disabilities, and some researchers, have explored the nuances of ethical concerns.

Access

Despite these general safeguards, other ethical issues may arise during the design or implementation of research with a vulnerable population. The first issue is gaining access to the research site. A 'gatekeeper' is a person or group who determines who may access a particular setting and the people for whom they are responsible, and how. The gatekeeper may have conflicting allegiances: for example, a hospital administrator may desire the prestige and eventual benefits of research but must also protect psychiatric patients from interactions that may impede their recovery. Accessing the research site began with a suggestion from a thesis committee member that I contact the board and care home owners, whom he knew. I sent a letter outlining the research to the home administrator and discussed my project fully during a subsequent interview. Although his support was received directly, the process of final approval was decided by the residents at their monthly house meeting. I heard no negative reactions to the proposed research and obtained approval from the residents via the administrator.

Power relations

Although the process of approval seemed democratic, I wondered if all 50 residents truly approved of my presence and research goals. Symptoms associated with the illnesses of many residents included apathy, lack of assertiveness and disorganized thinking. These symptoms may have interfered with their

ability to articulate a protest, or even to ask questions. Just as important was the inherent power differential between the residents and the management and, by association, myself. In addition to giving up some amount of agreed-upon control to the management, the residents with chronic mental illnesses are a marginalized group in society. Such marginalization, and other factors, contributes to feelings of disem-powerment and actions consistent with those feelings. My lack of response to this ethical concern was influenced by a perceived need to meet a rapidly approaching deadline for completion of the research. The belief that I would behave respectfully towards all residents, and be particularly sensitive to issues of privacy and autonomy, lessened my immediate concerns. Considerable thought and negotiation are necessary to conduct research to the highest ethical standard, meet research goals and, for many researchers, acknowledge the career benefits of funded research and publication. These issues remain problematic for researchers whose potential participants have difficulty confronting an authority figure, and who may possibly refuse to participate.

Informed consent

Many of the same concerns stated above are relevant to obtaining the informed consent necessary for residents to participate in the research. Five participants I approached seemed to read the consent form carefully, as evidenced by their questions. One person found the 'degree of risk' explanation rather amusing: 'You may feel some discomfort or dissatisfaction regarding the researcher's questions or her presence' (Suto 1988). Two people did not appear to read the form and another person asked me to read it to her, which I did. Again, questions of disempowerment and symptom interference could have been explored further. The development of a consent form that meets the requirements of an ethical review board and is user-friendly for participants who may have some cognitive dysfunction, is also challenging.

Symptom interference

Individuals with chronic schizophrenia may have symptoms that interfere with accurate representations of their experiences. This cannot always be identified prior to starting the research, nor would it be a valid reason not to gather data from individuals with illnesses such as schizophrenia. In this project there were inconsistencies in data from particular individuals, such as Rosemary's difficulty in recalling her hospitalizations. Triangulation of data sources and methods addresses this problem adequately. For example, during an interview a participant describes social activities or patterns of television viewing: participant observation at the sites of her reported activities provides one opportunity to confirm these data; asking other residents or staff is another effective strategy. The kinds of inaccuracies I suspected but was unable to confirm often involved less important data, such as age, hospitalizations, work history and family constellation. These uncertainties did not impede an effective analysis of the environment and residents' time use.

Concerns about symptom interference and consistency of data reinforce the choice of multiple data collection methods for this population and others with similar vulnerabilities. Participant observation requires researchers to develop a good memory for detail. Writing highly descriptive field notes instead of glossing over data or making premature inferences is far more important than participants' occasional inconsistencies in reporting their thoughts, feelings or behaviours. Analysis and sufficient time in the field should mitigate the effects of symptoms and inaccurate renditions of events.

Impact of the researcher's presence

The research setting is often a new environment for the researcher, which challenges them to search carefully for evidence of their influence on the milieu. In the initial research design phase, I anticipated that my presence in the board and care home might affect the research findings adversely. First was the issue of my presence on the natural flow of conversation, events and behaviours. Admittedly I was a new face at the facility, and had a different role from residents or staff. The ratio of researcher to residents and my interpersonal approach limited the influence my presence had on the milieu. It is difficult to determine whether and how conversations were edited in my presence. Residents often acknowledged me by making eye contact, saying hello, nodding to me or starting a conversation. They seemed often to continue with whatever they were doing, unless conversation subsequently ensued.

Secondly, I wondered whether my presence would elicit obvious impression management or attempts 'to pass', that is, concealing information about oneself to avoid being regarded as anything but 'normal' (Goffman 1963, p. 74). Many people were candid with me about their psychiatric histories, lack of family support and limited job prospects. Neither the content of the data nor the residents' behaviour that I observed suggested substantial adaptation to my presence. Thirdly, participant observation and interviews had the potential to disrupt facility or personal routines. As there was a considerable amount of unstructured time, the duration of interviews did not seem to interfere unduly with residents' activities. In summary, actions that might have compromised the residents' privacy or significantly altered their customary participation within the setting were monitored and, for the most part, avoided. The critical mass of residents seemed to serve as some protection against the potential impact of my presence on either the home or the research findings.

CONCLUSION

Data collection concerns for qualitative research projects focusing on vulnerable participants form the basis of this chapter. Examples of the advantages and disadvantages of participant observation, ethnographic interviews and document review were drawn from a research project conducted with a marginalized group: people with chronic mental illnesses. Various criticisms of each data collection method notwithstanding, obtaining data from a number of sources over a prolonged period of time enhanced the rigour of the study. Ethical concerns of the kind that are likely to arise in qualitative research with people who have chronic schizophrenia must be anticipated in the research design phase, and also negotiated during the data collection period. Qualitative methods remain an appropriate choice for understanding the kinds of complex challenges of daily living that face people with chronic mental illnesses.

REFERENCES

American Psychiatric Association 1987 Diagnostic and statistical manual of mental disorders. American Psychiatric Association, Washington, DC

Atkinson P, Hammersley M 1994 Ethnography and participant observation. In: Denzin NK, Lincoln YS (eds) Handbook of qualitative research. Sage, Thousand Oaks, CA, pp 248–261

Bogdan RC, Biklen SK 1998 Qualitative research for education: an introduction to theory and methods, 3rd edn. Allyn & Bacon, Boston

Emerson RM, Fretz RI, Shaw LL 1995 Writing ethnographic fieldnotes. University of Chicago, Chicago, IL

Fontana A, Frey JH 1994 Interviewing: the art of science. In: Denzin NK, Lincoln YS (eds) Handbook of qualitative research. Sage, Thousand Oaks, CA, pp 361–376

Goffman E 1963 Stigma: notes on the management of spoiled identity. Prentice-Hall, Englewood Cliffs, NJ

Janesick VJ 1994 The dance of qualitative research design. In: Denzin NK, Lincoln YS (eds) Handbook of qualitative research. Sage, Thousand Oaks, CA, pp 209–219

Krefting L 1991 Rigor in qualitative research: the assessment of trustworthiness. American Journal of Occupational Therapy 45(3):214–222

Suto M 1988 A study of future-time perspective in individuals with chronic schizophrenia. Unpublished Master's thesis, University of Southern California, Los Angeles

Suto M, Frank G 1994 Future time perspective and daily occupations of persons with chronic schizophrenia in a board and care home. American Journal of Occupational Therapy 48(1):7–18

FURTHER READING

Emerson H, Cook J, Polatajko H, Segal R 1998 Enjoyment experiences as described by persons with schizophrenia: a qualitative study. Canadian Journal of Occupational Therapy 65(4):183–192

Estroff S 1981 Making it crazy: an ethnography of psychiatric clients in an American community. University of California, Berkeley, CA

Rebeiro KL, Allen J 1998 Voluntarism as occupation. Canadian Journal of Occupational Therapy 65:279–285

Spradley JP 1979 The ethnographic interview. Holt, Rinehart & Winston, New York

5

Client–partner relationships post stroke: exploring the perspectives of couples

Sue Stanton

KEY POINTS

identifying and recruiting participants; theoretical sampling; interviewing couples: developing interview guides, setting up private interviews at home, gaining trust; researcher versus therapist role tension; tape recording; stroke

CHAPTER CONTENTS

OVERVIEW

This chapter focuses on the methodological issues inherent in a study that involves multiple participants focusing on participant sampling, interviewing family members and recording data during interviews. First, a synopsis of the research objectives and data collection is provided. Then, snapshots of the research process and findings related to one theme in the data, client–partner relationships, illustrate the key points. Problems that arose in these areas and how they were addressed are discussed. A summary of the research findings and implications, and the potential contributions of this type of research to the delivery of client-centred health services, conclude the chapter.

BACKGROUND TO THE STUDY

Rehabilitation professionals frequently come into contact with immediate family members when making arrangements for clients to be discharged home and providing community-based services. Even so, the focus of rehabilitation is typically on the person who has had the stroke. Once discharged from health services, the day-to-day experiences of former clients and their immediate family members become invisible. Has the rehabilitation process prepared them for this transition? Do they know where to find the resources they may need? How do their relationships change? How do they adapt to the change in life path and role that is often triggered by residual disability post stroke? It was these types of questions that led to a qualitative study exploring the process of adaptation at home (up to 31 months post stroke), from the perspective of individuals who had experienced a stroke and of their partners.

RESEARCH OBJECTIVES

The study aimed to describe and analyse the process of adaptation, both for the person who had had the stroke and for their partner, and to develop a theory of adaptation over time post stroke. Specific objectives included examining:

- participants' beliefs and explanations about the stroke, and how they changed over time
- participants' experiences of the problems the stroke caused, how they coped with them, and how this changed over time
- how the stroke affected roles, friendships and family relationships, and how these changed over time
- the impact of the environment on adaptation over time, and
- the impact of the stroke on the life of partners over time.

DATA COLLECTION

Data for the study were drawn from in-depth semi-structured interviews, observations of participants during the interviews, and from medical data obtained by the occupational therapist who recruited each person who had had a stroke. These 'medical' data included the client's age and gender, the date the stroke

occurred, the cerebral hemisphere in which it occurred and, if available, the cause of the cerebrovascular accident (CVA).

The interviews were tape-recorded and transcribed, and data collection, coding and analysis proceeded jointly. Observations were also recorded. As the transcripts were reviewed, research team members identified emerging themes (the team comprised myself, the co-researcher Lyn Jongbloed, and a research assistant). Data were coded and categorized in ways that made sense of them (Hammersley & Atkinson 1995). Each research team member coded transcripts of interviews that she had conducted. A proportion were coded independently by two team members, and then checked and discussed to achieve consistency in categorization.

PARTICIPANT SAMPLING

The method of theoretical sampling described by Glaser and Strauss (1967) and Glaser (1978) was used in this study. Glaser (1978) defines *theoretical sampling* as 'the process of data collection for generating theory whereby the analyst jointly collects, codes, and analyzes his data and decides what data to collect next and where to find them, in order to develop his [sic] theory as it emerges' (p. 36). Thus, the need for information to aid the development of or substantiate emerging theory influences the decisions about the number of participants needed. Three aspects of the sampling method used in this study – identifying the targeted participants, recruiting participants, and the process of ongoing theoretical sampling from data – will be discussed in this section.

Identifying participants

For ongoing theoretical sampling from data to occur some data needed to be collected. As a starting point we consulted an experienced qualitative researcher, who advised us to seek 16–20 participants for the study, recognizing that more could be added later. Alternatively, if a theory was developed before all 20 had participated in all interviews, the amount of data sought could be decreased.

Given the study focus, it was logical for the data to be collected from people who had had a stroke, and their partners. Before locating and obtaining consent from participants, we needed to further define the desired participant characteristics. Would we, for example, include everyone who had had a stroke and had a living partner or spouse; those who did not speak English; those with aphasia; and those who could not answer our questions because of cognitive or other mental dysfunction? We asked these and other questions to identify criteria that would enable participants to play an active role in describing and exploring their experiences with the researchers.

The absence of longitudinal studies of post-stroke experiences and the anticipated volume of data the study would collect, indicated that narrowing the criteria would probably facilitate analysis of the data. A study by Morgan and Jongbloed (1990), for example, found that age and employment at the time of the stroke appeared to influence adjustment to stroke. So, initially we decided to include only people who had had a stroke who:

- had experienced a stroke 4–7 months prior to the study
- had no aphasia or cognitive impairment
- were 65 years of age or older
- were not employed at the time of the stroke
- had functional problems that limited participation in previous activities
- could communicate in English, and
- had a spouse/partner who was willing to participate in the study.

Recruiting participants

This proved to be a complex process that involved locating recruitment sites, obtaining site approvals, preparing site personnel and overcoming recruitment obstacles. Even though we wanted to explore participants' experiences after their discharge from rehabilitation programmes, we felt that waiting until then to identify potential participants would make recruitment a monumental task. Consequently, we approached two agencies that provided rehabilitation services after a stroke. We reasoned that the occupational therapists at each site would be in the best position to identify potential participants among their clients, to provide the baseline health record information and, in consultation with the researchers, determine whether the other criteria were met.

Obtaining site approvals

Before recruitment could begin, the research committee at each site reviewed the project. In some cases a separate ethics review form and cover letter were submitted; in others a cover letter and copies of the completed University Ethics Review Form and Ethics Approval notification were sufficient. All of this took time. This process was required even though the data collection did not commence until after discharge.

It was also agreed that the primary agency contact person for the study would be compensated from the research grant for recruitment time. Some agencies, however, would not allow direct payment to this person even when they worked overtime on the recruitment tasks, perceiving that they had done so during the time they were paid by the agency.

Preparing site personnel and recruiting participants

Once ethics approval at each site was received, one occupational therapist was chosen as the contact person to enhance communication with the researchers, and to ensure that the same information was provided to all potential participants and that recruitment procedures were followed. The orientation provided by one of the researchers for each contact person included recruitment criteria, how to approach potential participants, and the process for gaining consent from each client and their partner. Separate consents were obtained from clients and partners: only when both consented were they considered to be research participants.

A research assistant acted as the primary project liaison person for the researchers. She was responsible for answering any questions, reorientating contact people when necessary, monitoring the progress of recruitment, ensuring that the consent procedures were followed, and following up with each agency when recruitment was not occurring.

Overcoming recruitment obstacles

Identifying sufficient participants who met the criteria was a challenge, but the last criterion proved to be most troublesome: although there was no shortage of people who had had a stroke, the partners of many had died. This was particularly true for women who had had a stroke and were younger than their spouse. Not having a researcher at each site also slowed recruitment. The most important role of the site personnel was to provide occupational therapy services to clients: consequently, recruitment of research participants for a study in which they were not investigators inevitably had a lower priority. Several changes to the recruitment strategy were made to enhance recruitment. These included:

- changing criteria: the age limit was lowered to 55 years to increase the chance that the stroke survivor had a living spouse or partner; and the partner was redefined to include non-partner primary household members who had lived in the same dwelling for at least 5 years, shared household work and socialized with each other
- adding three more recruitment sites, and the contact people at each site
- increasing site visits and telephone follow-ups to check recruitment progress, and
- advising the contact people at the first two sites of the changes in criteria.

Even with these changes it took 18 months to recruit 20 participants. A profile of these participants is provided in Table 5.1.

Suggestions to enhance the initial recruitment process are noted in Box 5.1

Table 5.1 Profile of participants

Number of participants and their relationship: $n = 40$
(20 persons with stroke)
   18 couples were married
   1 pair was a parent and son
   1 pair was two men

Participants with stroke
   Age range 55–80 years
      Mean = 67 years
      SD = 6.73
   15 men and 5 women
   11 had left hemiplegia, 9 right hemiplegia

Length of hospital (inpatient) stay
   Range 1–27 weeks
   Mean = 12.23
   SD = 7.57

Barthel scores (Client scores on the Mini-Mental Status Test [Folstein et al 1975] and the Barthel Index [Mahoney & Barthel 1965] were used as criteria for participation in the study)
   Range 55–100
   Mean = 86.5
   SD = 10.53

THEORETICAL SAMPLING FROM DATA

Glaser (1978) and Strauss and Corbin (1990) provide rich, detailed descriptions of the process of theoretical sampling through coding and analysing the data. Three types of increasingly specific coding, (a) open, (b) axial and (c) selective, directed the sampling process. *Open coding* begins the process by breaking down

---

Box 5.1 Suggestions to enhance initial recruitment of participants

- Carefully consider the ways to identify participants; use available networks.
- Allow time for ethical approvals at each recruitment site, where such sites are needed.
- Ensure that there is designated funding to pay for recruiters at each site and 'protected time' for them to do this task.
- Monitor recruitment progress at regular intervals.
- Ensure your criteria are clear and well understood.
- Ensure that you only include criteria that are essential for collecting information, and ensure they are consistent with your research objectives.

data, comparing the pieces and identifying concepts, categories and subcategories. *Axial coding* explores and defines the relationship between the categories and subcategories, and in doing so begins the process of putting the data back together. Finally, in *selective coding* the 'core category' (or sometimes categories) is identified and integrated with the other categories to complete the theory. In each stage the analyst constantly compares data and categories for similarities and differences, going back to the data to verify theory at each stage of development. Thus, the theory that emerges is grounded in the data. The theoretical sensitivity of the researcher is crucial to theoretical sampling. Strauss and Corbin (1990) define *theoretical sensitivity* as the 'attribute of having insight, the ability to give meaning to data, the capacity to understand, and the capability to separate the pertinent from that which isn't' (p. 42). Simply put, it is the ability to see through the data to uncover underlying themes and develop concepts. It directs the researcher in identifying the need for more information to develop or substantiate emerging theory; that is, it directs theoretical sampling. Awareness of what is important in data and the ability to give them meaning comes from the researcher's personal and professional experience, and familiarity with

the literature (Strauss & Corbin 1990). It enables the researcher to see data in their concrete form as described by participants, and in other ways. An ability to see beyond the obvious and think in the abstract, both inductively and deductively, is a valuable analytical tool.

INTERVIEWING COUPLES

The interviews were the primary source of information about the participants' experiences after their or their partner's stroke. Interviewing members of the same household required two interview guides and careful planning in setting up interviews. It also brought some extra challenges in gaining participants' trust and ensuring confidentiality; and, for the interviewers, addressing the role tension that can occur when therapists are the researchers.

Developing interview guides

One of the first steps was to develop initial interview guides for the people who had had a stroke and their partners. The interview guides for a person with a stroke (Box 5.2) and for the partner (Box 5.3) were developed as a requirement for the Ethics Review, but they also helped the three interviewers to focus on the

---

Box 5.2 Interview guide for person who has had a stroke

Listed below are sample questions. Questions will not necessarily be asked in this order, or phrased in the way presented here.

I am interested in finding out what life has been like since your stroke. I think this will help us understand more about the difficulties strokes cause for people and how they cope with them.
- Tell me about your life since your stroke (or since I last spoke to you).
- What are the chief problems your stroke has caused for you during the last few months? (Ways of coping will be explored here.)
- How do you deal with problems that arise? (Different from before the stroke.)
- Could you describe a typical day?
- How is this different from a typical day before your stroke?
- What do you think caused your stroke?

- What is most important to you in your life now?
- What do you expect to be doing 5 years from now?
- What has been your chief fear since your stroke (or since I last spoke to you)?
- How has your stroke affected your relationship with your partner?
- How has your stroke affected your relationship with family members?
- How has the stroke affected your relationship with friends?

Questions and observations regarding:
- aspects of the environment that facilitate or hinder adjustment, e.g. transportation, location of shopping centre and community centre
- other medical or health conditions
- perception of support available and received.

> **Box 5.3** Interview guide for partner
>
> Listed below are sample questions. Questions will not necessarily be asked in this order, or phrased in the way presented here.
>
> I am interested in finding out what life has been like for you since your partner's stroke. I think that this will help us to understand more about the difficulties experienced by spouses/partners of individuals who have had a stroke and how they cope with these difficulties.
> - Tell me about your life since your partner's stroke (or since I last spoke with you).
> - What are the chief problems his/her stroke has caused for you during the last few months? (Ways of coping will be explored here.)
>
> - Could you describe a typical day to me?
> - How is this different from a typical day before your partner's stroke?
> - What do you think caused your partner's stroke?
> - What has been your chief fear since his/her stroke (or since I last spoke to you)?
> - How has your partner's stroke affected your relationship with him/her?
> - Could you tell me about particular people (or services) who/that have been supportive to you since your partner's stroke. (How the person experiences the relationship as supportive will be explored. Lack of social support and reasons for this will also be examined.)

same initial open-ended questions. Although the interviews were intended to be exploratory, it was necessary to provide some structure to focus the interviews because we anticipated up to 200 transcripts. Without structure it was less likely that the concepts could be harnessed sufficiently for theories to emerge in analysis, particularly early in the research. The literature review and professional experience informed the researchers about potential concepts that could be explored, and guided the development of the initial interview questions. As we did not want to prejudge the concepts that might emerge from the research, these were subject to change. Sticking rigidly to these questions through all the interviews would have constrained the theoretical sampling needed to generate theory. Our approach modelled the creative interviewing approach advocated by Douglas (1985), and we adapted ourselves to the participants' environments and their conversations.

Setting up the interviews

The two researchers and their assistant were assigned 'families' to interview. These remained constant throughout the study and enabled relationships between the interviewer and each 'family' to develop over time. Having one contact person for each family facilitated the communication needed to set up interview appointments and address any process issues

or concerns. Each interviewer set up their appointments ensuring that 2–3 hours were available to interview the 'client' and their partner, and that the time chosen was suitable for both.

Ensuring private space for interviews

Typically, before beginning the first interviews the participants identified who would be interviewed first and where each interview could be held privately within the home. In most cases this was straightforward, with interviews taking place in living or family room spaces, where a closed door to other rooms could provide privacy and ensure confidentiality for each interviewee. On two occasions participants challenged these arrangements, even though they had been advised that interviews would be separate.

One couple insisted on being interviewed together, saying that their views and ideas were similar. It was evident to the interviewer that if this did not happen, no interviews would take place. Although the interviews proceeded, we recognized that this would need to be considered during the analysis. The woman, who had experienced the stroke, appeared to take the lead role and responded to the majority of questions. Her husband participated much less, even with the probing, open interview style used. The interviewer believes that even if this man had been interviewed alone, his responses would not have been greater. The participation of this couple ceased after the third interview because no new information was being elicited.

An incident occurred in the first interviews with another couple. I had completed the interview of the man, who had had the stroke, when an altercation occurred prior to his wife's interview. The man objected to his wife being interviewed privately, saying that she would say nasty things about him. He seemed very agitated and began to raise his 'quad cane' (walking stick) in the air, as if to strike her. I intervened and explained that private interviews were a research requirement. The explanation seemed to resolve the situation; he returned to the kitchen and I commenced the interview with his wife. This couple was interviewed five times over 2 years; there were no other threatening incidents of this nature.

Gaining trust

During the first interviews establishing rapport and gaining trust were significant issues, as rapport is a necessary prerequisite for trust. The participants needed to feel that we understood them and were willing to attempt to see the situations they experienced from their perspectives. It was also important that they felt comfortable enough with the interviewer to tell their stories, express their feelings, and raise issues of importance to them.

A time for testing

Part of the process in the first interview was discussing the general format and recording of the interview and confirming, as noted on their consent form, that participants did not have to answer questions and could withdraw from the study at any time. During these interviews I was very conscious that participants were 'checking me out'. Although they could end the interviews at any time, the first one seemed the most likely time for that to occur. If they had not wished to continue, that would have meant the loss of two participants, which was a concern as recruitment had been such a challenge. I was very attentive

to the surroundings, showing respect for their environment as a visitor and responding to their cues regarding discomfort, time, and offers of tea. Some participants maintained a very formal environment, others invited me to have tea with them before or during the interview; this seemed like a more natural part of being in a visitor role, and broke the tension.

Enhancing trust

The nature of the interviewer's questions and responses can convey an understanding of the participant's situation that facilitates the development of trust. In the following example the researcher has reworded the partner's first comment without changing the main message. In doing so, she creates the impression that she is validating the partner's comment. This type of comment builds trust and helps the participant (P) to feel comfortable with the interviewer (I).

P: That's not easy work, playing squash.
I: No, it's quite demanding.
P: That's right. And in a tournament you want to do your best so you push yourself and he will push himself that way.

During the course of the interviews the climate changed. As the interviewers and participants became more comfortable with each other, the tone of the interviews was more relaxed and natural, and the participants appeared more willing to reveal stories and experiences about their everyday lives.

Providing reassurance

Some hesitancy to participate in the first interview was evident for some participants, as noted in the section on private interviews. Occasionally, 'partner' participants remarked that they did not want their comments shared with the partner who had had the stroke. This occurred even though all participants had been advised that their responses would be treated confidentially and that their names would not be included in any reports associated with the research. Reassurance appeared to resolve their concerns. Two other partners also requested reassurance related to 'being correct'. Early in the first interview one partner said that she was not sure whether she should participate because she did not know if she could provide the 'right' information. I reassured her that since we were asking people to describe their own experiences, any of her responses would be 'right' for us. Another partner needed reassurance about whether she was managing her husband's stroke 'in the right way'. I gave a similar response the first time this occurred; however, in the second interview it became clear that this comment had not satisfied her completely. This time, I responded by saying that she had provided many suggestions for coping that I suspected others in the same situation would find innovative and helpful. By focusing on how the information she was sharing could benefit others in the future, rather than saying she was doing 'the right things', I indirectly validated her efforts. She did not raise this issue again.

Researcher versus therapist role tension

As interviewers we became aware of difficulties in couples' relationships. These were more evident in the second and third interviews, when it was becoming more apparent that the partner with the stroke might not recover completely, but in some cases they were still present in the last interviews. At times direct conflict was observed, whereas at other times the conflicts were described during the interviews. Disagreements were diverse. They included arguments about financial management, moving to an apartment, getting assistance, changes in roles, respite care, exercise programmes, activity (or the lack of it) by the person who had had the stroke, and dangerous driving. The following example involving a woman who had had a stroke shortly after her husband's retirement, when they had expected to be doing a lot of travelling, illustrates the type of tension experienced by the interviewers:

(Name of husband) and I have been having a real bad time lately – we're not getting along, we're at

each other and I know it's out of frustration. He doesn't blame me, but he can't help thinking, if it wasn't for me he'd be able to get on with his life. And with me I just feel guilt all the time, which I know I couldn't help it, so then we find we're snapping. I snap at him when I feel frustrated that I can't do things. Then he says, 'You're miserable to live with.' Which I am. But then he's no prize either, I tell him. And it starts, you know, the bickering, back and forth. And it's nobody's fault.

In some cases when observing these tensions we found ourselves wanting to recommend counselling. Being therapists sometimes made us feel that we should do something about the situation, but we knew it was important to keep the roles of therapist and researcher distinct. Consequently, we consciously re-directed questions to ask participants about how they managed the situation and what they thought might help them resolve their difficulties. Most participants discovered their own solutions over time.

The interview profile

Each participant was visited at home up to five times over a 2-year period. With one exception, each visit consisted of two interviews: one with the individual who had experienced a stroke, and one with the partner. All interviews were tape-recorded. Five couples were interviewed five times over 2 years, 13 couples were interviewed four times, one couple was interviewed three times, and one couple was interviewed twice. Those who were interviewed less than five times had generally regained stability in their lives following the stroke at the time of their last interviews, and so further interviews were considered redundant. The first interviews occurred between 4 and 7 months after the onset of the stroke and the remainder were spaced over the 2 years. Altogether 164 interviews were conducted.

RECORDING DATA IN THE INTERVIEWS
Tape-recording

We believed that the most effective way to document participants' experiences accurately was through tape-recording. Other advantages of tape-recording include:

• The interview can proceed as naturally as possible.

• The interviewer can make supplementary field notes without interrupting the flow of conversation and with the assurance that, once checked, the conversation is being recorded.

• The conversation is not being filtered and interpreted by the researcher as it occurs.

• Interviewers can give their full attention to the conversation. In so doing listening is enhanced and, as Strauss and Corbin (1990) suggest, adjustments can be made to questions during the interview. In this way questions or issues the interviewer planned to explore can be dropped or be supplemented 'on the spot'. If the interviewer is skilled, the end result is richer, denser and more meaningful data.

There are several potential disadvantages to tape-recording that require management strategies:

• The tape recorder can malfunction, leading to a loss of data, and so to minimize this possibility the functioning of the tape recorder needs to be checked every time it is used. We used a tape-recorder with a recording light so that when it was in view it could be unobtrusively checked to see whether the tape was moving. I also carried a back-up mini-tape recorder that would have sufficed in the event of a failure.

• The microphone may not pick up the conversation well enough for accurate transcription. We used a large conference microphone that looked unconventional. It was a flat, thin piece of steel approximately 5″ square: it was unobtrusive, multidirectional and very reliable.

• Much time needs to be allocated for the transcription of the interviews.

• Each transcript needs to be checked for accuracy. In this study each interviewer attempted to fill in any gaps that the secretary could not decipher because of a client's accent or dysphasia. Occasionally, words or phrases were lost because they could not be understood.

FINDINGS

Adaptation to stroke is a multifaceted process and the actions of each person in a relationship can have a huge impact on the adaptation of the other. All clients in the study received rehabilitation services post stroke; however, it was upon returning home that the real work of adaptation began. Although there were recurring themes in the data, each phase – 'transition', 'venturing out' and 'on the level' – in the journey towards 'normality' after the stroke had unique features with respect to client–partner relationships.

The *transition* phase occurred as the clients and partners made adjustments after discharge home. Here, daily life focused on carrying out self-care tasks and establishing a new routine that matched the client's capabilities. Strain and physical exhaustion were often present, and disagreements occurred about how to provide assistance and what and how much the client could do. Even so, there was a sense that this would pass once physical function improved. Once the couple was comfortable with routines and self-care tasks at home, they began *venturing out*. Visiting friends, relatives and Stroke Clubs; resuming sports and other leisure activities in the community; doing yard-work and driving were some of the occupations explored and tested. Here the couple came face to face with the limitations of disability on their anticipated future. While the couple attempted to negotiate new roles, make decisions and solve problems, each person was also coming to terms with the changes the disability brought to their roles, lifestyle and personal vision for the future. The 'biographical work' (Corbin & Strauss 1991) associated with such changes compounded the day-to-day irritations and frustrations in managing life after the stroke.

In time, the focus on exploration and experimentation diminished and the daily lives of couples appeared to be *on the level*. Here, clients and partners were likely to describe their lives as normal. Although their activities may have been different from before the stroke, they had a sense of what was possible, what methods contributed most to success, and what community resources were most helpful. Although they may not have been happy with their situation, there was greater stability in their lives.

Recurring themes through all phases

The road back to a more stable life was fraught with challenges for both clients and partners. Two recurring conditions appeared to have an ongoing influence on adaptation: role strain and physical exhaustion, and the quality of the relationship. Exhaustion was common as clients worked to regain physical function and resume valued occupations. Likewise, partners were exhausted from the added responsibilities associated with new roles (Jongbloed et al 1993). The strain of new and added partner roles parallels the findings of other research on chronic illness (e.g. Power 1985, Corbin & Strauss 1988, Charmaz 1991, Anderson 1992, Dale et al 1997).

Analysis of the data also revealed two distinct patterns in client–partner relationships: one facilitated adaptation post stroke, and the another constrained it. Couples with facilitating relationships were more likely to report having close relationships both pre and post stroke, sharing interests and household management, and communicating to share feelings and solve problems. These partners encouraged, coached and supported the client in resuming their chosen activities. Similarly, clients coached their partners in learning new roles, such as financial management and home repairs, and also supported their continued participation in valued past activities. Although frustrated and irritated at times, they used their communication skills to resolve differences.

In contrast, couples in constraining relationships often reported feeling frustrated and irritable, and were less able to communicate to solve problems or create joint goals. Although rare among facilitating couples, the partners in constraining couples were more likely to assume the parent-like role of 'gatekeeper' by discouraging or preventing their partner from attempting an activity. Although fear of injury from a fall initially sparked such action, after a while it became a pattern that reduced the client's motivation to participate in valued activities, akin to the learned helplessness described by Seligman (1975). Such clients often reported feelings of irritability and depression.

Two-thirds of the couples in this study tended to have relationships that were more facilitating, whereas one-third were more constraining. The quality of the couple's relationship appeared to have a greater impact on adaptation post stroke than individual responses to the stroke, or the extent of physical disability. This result is comparable to the findings of Corbin and Strauss (1984, 1988) and Power (1985).

IMPLICATIONS FOR PRACTICE

These findings illustrate the interdependence of family members, and the influence that clients' adaptation to disability at home following a stroke has on partners, and vice versa. An emphasis on physical recovery and the management of self-care tasks in rehabilitation appears to be insufficient to facilitate the achievement of clients' goals. Access to rehabilitation services in the client's home and community environment, up to 3 years post stroke, may help clients and partners to resolve the differences that limit resumption of past activities, and to explore and develop new skills that not only enhance adaptation but also improve quality of life. As Hammell (1998) points out, 'models of service delivery should enable responsive professional support in the community as new problems are encountered or the need for new skills and equipment is identified' (p. 132). Combined with information about community resources and respite for partners who need it, these services may break the downward cycle that can lead to partner exhaustion and depression, and low participation in valued activities for both clients and partners.

Today, evidence-based practice is considered essential in health care. Egan et al (1998) indicate that this term 'refers to the formulation of treatment decision using the best available research evidence' (p. 136). Health providers are expected to draw upon the most credible research findings and expert opinion to guide their decision making. Typically, however, quantitative research that emphasizes physical techniques has received greater recognition as a resource for rehabilitation practice. Although it has value, such research rarely provides the rich, in-depth information about the social world of people with disabilities and their families that can be gained from qualitative research. Occupational and physical therapists consider the clients' social world when working with them to achieve goals, and so the use of such knowledge has the potential to redefine best practice in rehabilitation by:

- expanding therapists' understanding of the day-to-day lives of people with disabilities and their families
- providing knowledge about approaches and resources that may contribute to the resolution of the potential or actual problems the client and family face once the client returns home
- guiding therapists' reasoning and questioning during the occupational or physical therapy process, so that practice reflects professional theories, and
- assisting therapists to create services that will enable people to live meaningfully in their communities and achieve their goals for participation in self-care, productivity or leisure occupations.

Acknowledgements

Dr Lyn Jongbloed was a co-investigator in the early stages of this research project; her participation and assistance was much appreciated. Barbara Fousek was the research assistant. Funding for this study was provided by the British Columbia Health Research Foundation.

REFERENCES

Anderson R 1992 The aftermath of stroke: the experience of patients and their families. Cambridge University Press, Cambridge

Charmaz K 1991 Good days, bad days: the self in chronic illness and time. Rutgers University Press, New Brunswick

Corbin J, Strauss AT 1984 Collaboration: couples working together to manage illness. Image: The Journal of Nursing Scholarship 15(4):109–115

Corbin J, Strauss AT 1988 Unending work and care: managing chronic illness at home. Jossey-Bass, San Francisco

Corbin J, Strauss A 1991 Comeback: the process of overcoming disability. Advances in Medical Sociology 2:137–159

Dale L, Gallant M, Kilbride L et al 1997 Stroke caregivers: do they feel prepared? Occupational Therapy in Health Care 11(1):39–53

Douglas JD 1985 Creative interviewing. Sage, Beverly Hills

Egan M, Dubouloz CJ, VonZweck C, Vallerand J 1998 The client-centred evidence-based practice of occupational therapy. Canadian Journal of Occupational Therapy 65(3):136–143

Folstein MF, Folstein SE, McHugh PR 1975 Mini-mental state: a practical method for grading the cognitive state of patients for the clinician. Journal of Psychiatric Research 12:189–198

Glaser B 1978 Theoretical sensitivity. Sociology Press, Mill Valley, CA

Glaser BG, Strauss AT 1967 The discovery of grounded theory: strategies for qualitative research. Aldine, Chicago

Hammell KW 1998 Client-centred occupational therapy: collaborative planning, accountable intervention. In: Law M (ed) Client-centred occupational therapy. Slack, Thorofare, pp 123–143

Hammersley M, Atkinson P 1995 Ethnography: principles in practice. Routledge, London

Jongbloed L, Stanton S, Fousek B 1993 Family adaptation to altered roles following a stroke. Canadian Journal of Occupational Therapy 60(2):70–77

Mahoney EK, Barthel EW 1965 Functional evaluation: the Barthel Index. Maryland State Medical Journal 14:61–65

Morgan D, Jongbloed L 1990 Factors influencing leisure activities following a stroke: an exploratory study. Canadian Journal of Occupational Therapy 57(4):223–229

Power PW 1985 Family coping behaviours in chronic illness: a rehabilitation perspective. Rehabilitation Literature 46:78–83

Seligman M 1975 Helplessness: on depression, development and death. WH Freeman, San Francisco

Strauss AT, Corbin J 1990 Basics of qualitative research: grounded theory procedures and techniques. Sage, Newbury Park

FURTHER READING

Becker G 1993 Continuity after a stroke: implications of life-course disruption in old age. Gerontologist 33(2):148–158

Hammersley M, Atkinson P 1995 Ethnography: principles in practice, 2nd edn. Routledge, London

Hasselkus BR 1990 Ethnographic interviewing: a tool for practice with family caregivers for the elderly. Occupational Therapy Practice 2(1):9–16

Jongbloed L 1994 Adaptation to a stroke: the experience of one couple. American Journal of Occupational Therapy 48(11):1006–1013

6

Representation and accountability in qualitative research

Karen Hammell

OVERVIEW

This chapter looks at a study that sought to explore perceptions of quality of life among people with high spinal cord injuries. The central theme of the chapter concerns the social relations of research and accountability to study participants, posing the question: 'Who do we want to value our research?' The chapter considers issues of power and knowledge, contemplating how the cooperative and collaborative process of qualitative research may be respected at all stages of data collection, analysis, writing and publication.

INTRODUCING THE STUDY: THE FORESHADOWED PROBLEM AND 'MEASURING' QUALITY

Little research has attempted to determine whether people who are paralysed below the neck following high spinal cord injury feel satisfied with survival and their subsequent lives. However, confronted with high spinal cord-injured survivors in both my personal and my professional life, I had become fascinated by two fundamental questions which became the basis for my subsequent doctoral research: Is a meaningful life possible after high spinal cord injury? And, if so, what *kind* of life is possible?

High spinal cord injury refers to the most severe form of spinal cord lesion that results from damage to the cervical nerves C1–C4, high in the neck. The term *high lesion tetraplegia* (formerly known in North America as quadriplegia) is used to describe the profound neurological deficit caused by this damage and which results in complete loss of motor and sensory function below the shoulders. People with spinal cord injuries at C3 or C4 may be able to breathe independently using solely their diaphragms, but those with injuries at C1 or C2 will almost certainly be dependent upon a ventilator for respiratory support. In addition, virtually every physiological system of the body will be affected by a high cord lesion. But what of the subsequent quality of life?

I suggest that the idea of 'measuring' quality should best be considered an oxymoron; none the less, there is an evident preoccupation among researchers with trying to quantify the inherently qualitative. Two contradictory views underpin contemporary definitions of quality of life. As Roy (1992) claims, 'the expression "quality of life" refers both to the experiences that make life meaningful and to the conditions that allow people to have such experiences' (p. 3). The inherent problem with quality of life assessment therefore involves the philosophical discrepancy between the *experience of meaningful life* and *life conditions*.

SELECTING A RESEARCH METHODOLOGY: THE CASE FOR QUALITATIVE RESEARCH

In reviewing the literature it became evident that so little was known about the lived experience of high tetraplegia that an exploratory, qualitative approach to the study was the only legitimate means by which to generate information (Bogdan & Biklen 1998).

Clearly, the choice of a research methodology should be informed by the nature of the problem it seeks to address. I believed that qualitative methodologies had a clear fit with the nature of the problem I had identified for research: examining 'quality'.

When I discussed my research with Alan, one of the study participants (all names have been changed to preserve anonymity), I told him about Gerhart et al's (1994) study in which the researchers determined that only 18% of emergency care providers would wish to be alive with a severe spinal cord injury. He responded: 'I'm surprised it was that many!' He expressed to me his belief that health-care professionals need to know more about what sort of life is possible following high spinal cord injury: 'And it has to be from us, in our voices'. The mandate to pursue a qualitative study could scarcely have been more clear.

RESEARCH AND POWER

Disability activists are forcing researchers to reflect upon the implications of the inevitable power imbalance between those who do research and those who are researched. Oliver (1997) argues that disabled people have come to see research as a violation of their experience and as irrelevant to their needs – in fact, 'nothing more than a "rip-off"' (p. 15). Indeed, he suggests that 'much research on disability has contributed little or nothing to improving the quality of life of disabled people, though it might have substantially improved the career prospects of the researchers' (Oliver 1987, p. 10). Further, he claims that because most researchers have little regular contact with disabled people the social relations of research remain the same, whether the chosen methodology is quantitative or qualitative: a case of changing the rules but not the game (Oliver 1992).

This position is echoed by Ward and Flynn (1994), who claim that when relatively powerful *'experts'* carry out research on relatively powerless *subjects*, the social relations of research do not change simply because a qualitative research methodology is used, 'despite the liberal trappings of the qualitative paradigm' (p. 31). Such claims demand that all researchers make a self-conscious scrutiny of what they study, why they are studying and who is to benefit from the research. This self-reflection must extend to the social relations of research, striving for collaborative relationships at every stage of the process.

RESEARCH PLANNING: RESPECT AND COLLABORATION

All research, regardless of the selected approach, depends upon the goodwill of those whose informed consent assures the researcher of a degree of cooperation. In addition, much qualitative research strives for a level of collaboration that places people and politics at the centre of the research endeavour.

In my own study I was reluctant to request any unwarranted intrusion into the lives of the study participants or to place unreasonable demands upon their time, yet I wished to achieve a high degree of collaboration with them: a position that influenced the design of my study.

Initially, I discussed my proposed research with a friend and colleague who has many contacts – and a considerable reputation – among the spinal cord-injured community. She, in turn, approached three people with high spinal cord injuries and explained to them my background and the aims of the study. They all agreed to their names and addresses being given to me so that I could contact them in person.

One of these three people is a vibrant force among the community of people with high lesion tetraplegia and was clearly going to be both a key informant and someone who could

facilitate my access to other potential participants. It was important to me to establish my authenticity as a researcher and to avoid the perception of being exploitative or parasitic. Accordingly, we arranged to meet so that I could explain my positioning in relation to the research, my perceived need for the study, what the research process would entail, and my intentions to share my doctoral thesis and research publications with those about whom I would write. He impressed upon me two concerns, which I incorporated into my planning for the research. One related to the discrepancy between society's view of high lesion tetraplegia and the reality of actually living with it (an impression that I shared); the other related to his perceived need to let people know there *is* life after spinal cord injury. He enthusiastically endorsed my study, promptly provided a list of several names of people he knew who would fit my stated criteria for participation, and when I thanked him profusely for his help and interest, told me: 'No, thank *you* for the study!' It was an encouraging beginning, and his sponsorship of both me and my study appeared to guarantee my welcome when I visited other participants.

Participant recruitment

From my initial contacts I used a 'snowball' method of sampling, through which participants suggested the names of other people who might be interested in participating (Bogdan & Biklen 1998). This method is commonly used by qualitative researchers as a means of gaining access to a certain population. It was hoped that it would ensure that all who participated would feel able to do so freely and willingly, rather than feeling compelled or obliged by having received initial contact through more formal channels.

A letter of introduction was sent to each potential participant, briefly explaining my background, my perceived need for the study and the anticipated process for conducting the research. It also included the following explanation:

I am concerned that the medical and rehabilitation professions, and indeed, the general public, know very little of what life is like for someone who has a high quadriplegia. My research therefore hopes to explore the issues which are pertinent to those who are already living with quadriplegia. It is my intention to publish my research findings in both the academic journals and the appropriate disability newsletters so that I am able to share what I have learned with all those who can best make use of the information in the future.

Fifteen men and women participated in the study: indeed, every one of the people whom I was able to contact agreed to participate (two other people were in hospital), which prompts consideration of whether I had a biased or 'élite' sample of people. A valid criticism of snowball sampling is that 'successful' people may suggest other 'successful' people, so that the sample is not representative of the group from which they are drawn. However, in light of the low prevalence of high spinal cord injury and my fairly restrictive inclusion criteria (especially in terms of geographic location, residency in the community – which stemmed from my desire to study 'possible' lives, by excluding those people who were confined to institutions, age and time since injury) I believe the 17 people whose names I received represent virtually the entire sample group from which they were drawn. I would therefore reject as logistically impossible the idea that I may have been steered towards a group of uniquely 'successful' people.

DATA COLLECTION

The interviewing process

The interview process was initially informed by a basic checklist of issues that arose from my own knowledge and experience, my familiarity with the academic and autobiographical literatures, and my desire to understand and document something of the lived experience of high lesion tetraplegia. By asking all 15 people to respond to the same topics I was able to compare themes across interview transcripts and identify member-generated issues and linkages. Thus, although the interviews were an evolving process and certain questions were dropped while other avenues of inquiry were explored in more depth (when I recognized their relevance and resonance for the participants), each participant was able to cover the same topics, and the last people I met were able to describe their experiences concerning each of my foreshadowed issues without being constrained by an increasingly narrow framework of inquiry (Box 6.1). I believed this would enable any discrepant views, differing opinions or contradictory interpretations to be identified and addressed.

Later, I returned to visit the first five participants for a second time and aimed to explore in more depth those topics that we had not previously examined in much detail, but which had emerged strongly from the study groups' stories. In an attempt to ensure that the

---

Box 6.1 Interview guide

- Can you tell me about your injury, in terms of what happened, how old you were and when it was?
- Could you tell me about life before your injury, what you were doing, what your interests were and so on?
- What did you initially think life would be like with a high spinal cord injury?
- Could you describe for me a typical day: where you go; what you do?
- Who provides your personal care assistance?
- Where has funding come from since your injury? (I don't want to know how much, just where it has come from.)

- How do you view your life now?
- [If positive!] What factors contribute to your satisfaction with life?
- What tends to make the bad days bad?
- What have been the most meaningful or significant events, or milestones in your life since your injury?
- Can you tell me about the experience of having control over your life?
- What is important to you in your everyday life?
- Are you involved with other disabled people? (Individually, or through organizations?)

interviews covered those aspects important to the participants (not solely those I had targeted for exploration), I always asked: 'Is there anything else I should have asked? Have I somehow missed the point?' This prompted responses such as 'What would I tell the world if I could?', followed by further thoughtful observations on the experience of living with high tetraplegia.

Positioning and politics

It is important to ponder how the research encounter was influenced by my social and personal positioning within it, examining how I, as the researcher, influenced and facilitated the cooperative and collaborative interaction that is fundamental to qualitative research.

It is accepted that the 'position' (gender, class, 'race', sexuality, age, religion, [dis]ablity and other dimensions of social differentiation) of the researcher will affect the research relationship and the nature of the data collected (see Chapters 1 and 10). However, I contend that as researchers of disability it is not sufficient to consider positionality as an equation of 'givens', but rather, we must consider our *chosen* positionality. As researchers, we make choices: Who will be our audience? Who do we wish to value our work? In a world inscribed by power, whose side are we on? Whose interests will be advanced through our research?

Perhaps it is not enough to state our personal and social positioning – where we are 'coming from' – but also our chosen political/philosophical positioning: where are we going *to*? These are factors that will serve to influence how we relate to our study participants, and whose purposes the knowledge will eventually serve.

Personal positioning

My personal positioning was clearly an integral part of the dynamics of my interactions with the participants. I was often asked for various forms of assistance: I moved arms and legs, wiped away tears, performed assistive coughs, and, most often, passed cups and positioned straws for the participants to sip at drinks during the

interviews. There was no apparent discomfort on the part of participants when a rattling leg bag was clearly audible, when a leg spasmed rhythmically, or when they discussed some of the more intrusive aspects of living with paralysis. My evident familiarity with the idiosyncrasies of this physical condition (owing to my husband's high spinal cord injury) clearly provided a level of comfort that encouraged the participants to ask me questions about my own life, to recruit my assistance with various care needs and to request my suggestions in identifying new equipment. This contributed to a level of reciprocity that I am persuaded – although not equalizing the power relations – reduced the distance between our inevitable dominant and subordinate positions. In addition, I suggest that my stated personal connection with the research topic may have contributed to the unusually high rate of participation in the study (100%).

I was very gratified by the unanimous cooperation I was given and the invitations that I subsequently received to attend meetings and social functions. The enthusiasm with which many of the participants agreed to participate, their universal willingness to entertain repeat interviews and the keen interest they have exhibited when I have chanced to encounter them in social and public contexts persuades me that the interviews had appeared relevant.

Philosophical/political positioning

Locating oneself as a positioned subject tends to pay respect to biographical axes of differentiation while failing to consider positioning from a political perspective. I have long believed that rehabilitation workers (clinicians as well as researchers) should align themselves with those upon whom their livelihood depends: disabled people. I suggest that our philosophical/political positionality will affect how disabled people see disability researchers: an issue of both credibility and authenticity.

Accordingly, I endeavoured to ensure that participants were aware that the research was not solely to be *about* people with high lesion tetraplegia: it aimed also to be *for* them, seeking to represent their priorities, agenda and viewpoints, using theoretical constructs that respected their humanity, providing a copy of my completed thesis and publishing the research findings in formats that would be accessible to disabled people (most particularly those with recent injuries).

Thus, I attempted to interpret data and theory in such a way that they would have resonance for those of whom I wrote. The study participants were not all academics, but they comprised intelligent people who were more than capable of recognizing a faithful representation and interpretation of their experience. It could therefore be claimed that my biographical positioning informed *why* I saw certain themes in my data; my philosophical positioning informed the theoretical perspective from which I interpreted those themes.

DATA ANALYSIS
Identifying themes

In qualitative research data analysis is not a distinct phase of the research but rather, begins prior to fieldwork, as research problems are formulated and clarified, and continues through the writing process. During the course of data collection I would document 'what am I getting?' and 'what am I not getting?', together with remarks such as 'I expected finance to be a big deal but it isn't', or 'how does occupation relate to life satisfaction?' This would help me to monitor my progress and identify the gaps in my understanding. Also, I wrote a line-by-line 'index' of each transcript, summarizing its content by a word or phrase, thereby creating a visual tally of the degree to which themes were repeated throughout our conversations.

Apart from unique (although none the less important) themes within each interview (such as details of a recent job interview, or past experiences of spousal abuse or cocaine addiction), I wished to include all of the data in my analysis and to try to account for linkages and associations between all themes,

not just certain themes. I was persuaded that my interviews all covered similar, interrelated material and concerned issues that were evidently linked in the minds of the participants, and that to work with certain themes at the expense of others would be to distort and misinterpret what I had been told.

Interpretation and theory

To interpret the stories of people's lives requires an imaginative process by which data are reduced to something manageable and cohesive. This is the role of theory. Acknowledging that there are numerous theoretical perspectives from which any study can be interpreted, I sought to judge the relative merits of various ones according to the degree to which they might be recognizable by members of the study population, might contribute to an understanding of the lived experience of disability that informs consideration of social policy issues, and might have resonance with theoretical perspectives proposed by disabled disability theorists. For example, I was reluctant to engage with some contemporary theories that reduce the experience of disability to clever metaphors or the construct of discourse: ideas that convey little respect and which are invariably couched in language that is inaccessible to the objects of theory. Further, I felt it to be important that the conceptual framework did not contain underlying normative judgements concerning 'superiority'/'inferiority', such as 'deviance', 'tragedy' or 'loss'. I was, however, strongly influenced by the concept of 'biographical disruption' (originally proposed by Bury 1982), for several reasons. Primarily, it made sense: describing the sudden disjuncture of a taken-for-granted life and reflecting both autobiographical accounts and my own clinical and personal experience. Further, it corresponded with the conceptual framework derived by disabled academics, who identified the dual notions of significant life events and biographical careers in a process they termed 'social adjustment' (Zarb et al 1990). In addition, biographical disruption enabled consideration of time use, in terms of everyday occupations, and of the temporal dimension of learning to live in an altered physical form, thereby incorporating theoretical perspectives from my own academic discipline of occupational therapy.

Although qualitative researchers often claim that theory emerges from empirical data (e.g. Morse 1994), it is apparent that it does so into a context of existing theoretical perspectives that are shaped in part by contemporary ideas (the intellectual 'climate') and in part by the personal philosophy and theoretical interests of the researcher. For this reason, Field and Morse (1985) indicate the need for the researcher 'to develop an acute sensitivity to the imbedded values and assumptions in society and in present day theories and research, and an acute self-awareness of one's own personal values, perspectives and biases' (p. 3).

Harris (1996) suggests that if researchers state clearly their personal locations and say, 'This is what I think is going on, here are the contradictions and complexities, from my point of view it could mean this' (p. 154), there is room for recognition that each analysis is but one of several possibilities. Harris argues that the principle of advocacy, as a political strategy, allows for the possibility that alternative interpretations can exist 'but that, politically, a strong case can be made for one's own' (p. 155).

Evaluating analyses

Sandelowski (1986) proposed that a qualitative study is credible or authentic 'when it presents such faithful descriptions or interpretations of a human experience that the people having that experience would immediately recognize it from those descriptions or interpretations as their own' (p. 30). It is worth considering whether disabled people – indeed all research participants – should be involved in the analysis and interpretation of data, perhaps providing informed consent for the consequent representation of their experiences. This would make the researcher responsible for articulating both language and explanations that could be readily understood by those outside the realms of intellectual élites, perhaps thereby ensuring a more relevant fit of analysis to data, and enhancing the possibility that members of the group under study could access and use the subsequent reports to advance their own causes. Once I had identified the themes and developed an interpretive framework, I returned to visit a participant who had already expressed an interest in helping me to determine the *authenticity* of my analysis (see Chapter 10). We spent a long time discussing the research; I would outline an interpretation and he would seek clarification or more detail. Finally, he declared himself 'very excited' about my work and found my proposed conceptual framework to be credible ('I *like* it!').

Ideally, I would have liked to include all 15 participants in the data analysis and interpretation. However, the prohibitive logistics and competing claims upon the participants' time and interests prevented me from requesting such a high level of commitment and from demanding further intrusion into their lives. The reality that I spent more time with one participant than with any other individual prompts consideration of whether I was, in some way, manipulated to convey a certain sort of narrative or pursue certain issues. Primarily, I suggest that if my study report presented descriptions that other people with high tetraplegia would recognize, then the issue of whose voice spoke the loudest may not be relevant. Further, I propose that his voice and perspectives provided a useful counterbalance to my own views, forcing me to explain and confront my own assumptions and to incorporate a different perspective into my thinking.

CONSTRUCTING THE WRITTEN TEXT
Seeing voices

In previous research that utilized a quantitative approach, I sought to understand the relationship between perceived levels of social support and levels of anxiety and depression among people with either severe closed head injury or spinal cord injury, and their partners. I used two research instruments that express a quantitative statement of these variables and which could be analysed statistically. In presenting my numerical findings, I was able to compare my data with those of other researchers and thereby question previously held assumptions about the uniqueness of the social isolation that had been reported by people with head injuries. However, the voices and perspectives of the 60 study participants were effectively silenced by this mode of presenting results.

In qualitative research efforts are made to record and re-present the words of the study participants. In my research into the experience of high tetraplegia, for example, I often asked what was it like to have lived for many years in an institution. A representative selection of the responses is presented here:

Well, I mean – *HELL* really – there was nothing I could compare it to … you sort of look back later on and ask, 'How'd I do it?' You know, 'How'd I get through it?' (David).

I wanted *to leave* the [long-term care] unit that I was in *SO BADLY* that … it became less important to me that I had a spinal cord injury than where I was (Beth).

I was kind of scared that I might be stuck in institutions for the rest of my life … and that was really scary because you had no freedom in there, no individuality, and you weren't really treated like a real person … it's just – a cesspool of humanity … and just seeing how other people are treated … a lot of them had speech impediments and can't really fend for themselves and they're really at the mercy of the staff (Luke).

The reason I'm living out of the [hospital] was to get out of that, uh, penitentiary feeling. They didn't need actual bars on the windows 'cause nobody was going to escape, but it was like a prison in every other sense (Owen).

Thus, in constructing the written text efforts are made to reflect and represent the voices and perspectives of the study participants, respecting their knowledge, opinions and viewpoints, and enabling the reader to determine the plausibility of the researcher's interpretations and conclusions.

Power and representation

Writing an account of qualitative research is a process of description and interpretation. The writer performs an 'act of translation', as a mediator between the research participant and the reader (Marcus & Fischer 1986, p. 31). Although efforts are made to present extracts from the interviews such that the actual words spoken by the participants are used in subsequent reports, it is important to acknowledge that the choice to present these words and not others reflects the choices and priorities of the researcher.

Although there is a significant body of literature addressing such issues within qualitative research as gaining access to research participants and of reflexivity during the interview process, far less attention has been paid to concerns of retaining the voices, perspectives and priorities of the participants in the phase of data analysis, writing up and subsequent publications (Edwards & Ribbens 1998).

Valuing knowledge

Traditionally, scientific knowledge was judged to be neutral, objective and value free, such that 'truths' might be determined. More recent recognition of the instability of claims to knowledge are reflected in the use of the null hypothesis in quantitative research, which states that relationships between variables may be disproved, but never proved with certainty. Despite contemporary intellectual recognition that all knowledge is inescapably shaped by social forces (e.g. economics, politics) and by the ideas and beliefs of the researchers, there remains within the literatures of medicine and rehabilitation an understated premise: that as clinicians and researchers *we* have knowledge, whereas our clients and research subjects have 'beliefs' (Good 1994). Good notes that 'knowledge requires certitude and correctness; belief implies uncertainty, error, or both' (p. 17). This élitist attitude obscures the realization that study participants might view things differently from the researcher, yet with *equal validity*

(Marcus & Fischer 1986). Qualitative research attempts to accord as much value to experiential knowledge (the lived experience of the study participants) as to the academic and practical knowledge of the researcher. This is congruent with the philosophy that underpins client-centred practice and with an ethics of respect.

ACCOUNTABILITY

Researchers in the quantitative tradition adhere to criteria that support the reliability and validity of their data and of their measurement tools. Chapter 10 will consider the criteria used by qualitative researchers to defend the rigour of their studies. However, I suggest that it is equally important to evaluate the impact of research on the disabled people we study. For example: Is the study important and relevant to the study participants? Would other people with similar disabilities immediately recognize the descriptions and interpretations as reflecting their own experiences? Who is to benefit from the research?

Moore, Beazley and Maelzer (1998) propose that 'the priority that *informants* attach to issues explored through any piece of disability research can be used as indices for gauging relevance and utility of the research findings' (p. 18). Further, they proposed that disability research should be reviewed critically in terms of its prospects for promoting disabled people's rights. This addresses accountability to research participants.

Evaluating research contributions

In reviewing my own research I believed it to have two potential contributions. First, by contributing to an understanding of how a group of severely disabled people see themselves, and thus by acknowledging the value of their lives (and that quality in living is possible for them), I hoped to contribute to challenging and changing attitudes that are grounded in 'ableist' values and normative judgements. Second, by examining *how* quality in life is attainable – beginning with the right to live autonomously in the community like other citizens – I hoped to contribute to challenging and changing social

policies that have confined severely physically disabled people in institutions.

I contend that these two aims, or claims, reflect the reasons the study participants gave for contributing to this research. Primarily, they stated that they wanted to let newly injured people – and society – know that there is life after high spinal cord injury, and that 'we are normal people just like everyone else'. For example, at the conclusion of our interview, Owen noted that my 'Informed Consent Form' had stated that I would destroy the recorded tapes at the completion of my research. He reiterated what all the participants had said – that he wished to do something to help people with recent injuries – and wanted me to keep the tape if his story would help someone: 'There's still so much to see and so much out there to appreciate … and if keeping this tape will help, I don't see any problem with hanging on to it. Hang on to it.' Further, several people spoke of the desire to see positive changes in social policy to facilitate community living for themselves and for other severely disabled people.

Throughout this project I was mindful of the observation that although research 'may lead to the compilation of a respectable academic PhD thesis … [it] can also mean that the work undertaken makes absolutely no positive, but plenty of negative, difference to those whose interests it claims to have at heart' (Moore et al 1998, p. 20). It has therefore been very rewarding to note the commitment the study participants showed to the research and its outcomes, by suggesting ways of promoting the findings with a view to bringing about changes in social attitudes and social policies. For example, one participant gave me a copy of a magazine produced by and for an advocacy group of disabled people in British Columbia, and asked me to promise to write about the study and submit this to the magazine (a commitment I am currently fulfilling). Another asked me to supply a copy of the final thesis to the spinal cord injury rehabilitation centre (which I have done); and several people raised the possibility that I should write a book about the study that would be accessible to 'the general public'.

I was consistently impressed by the apparent eagerness of many people to talk with me, the warm reception I received from all the participants, their assistants and family members, and the comments that were made about the interest or importance of the research itself. However, the observation that many people – 'other' people – value the opportunity to tell their stories should not, I believe, lead to complacency or smugness. I am persuaded that people with disabilities, including the participants in my own study, tell their stories, volunteer for medical or social science research, attend medical 'rounds' or complete questionnaires in the hope of helping others; and that this is part of finding meaning and purpose following an illness or injury. Thus, I understand their narratives to have been shared as part of a commitment to contributing to society – a theme recurring throughout the transcripts – rather than as a form of personal catharsis.

DISSEMINATING FINDINGS: USING KNOWLEDGE, SHARING POWER

Within academia knowledge is a commodity. Promotion, peer recognition and funding for further research is accorded through the accumulation of articles, books and papers in refereed journals, and conferences. Standing (1998) observes that the translation or interpretation of the spoken word into an academic presentation serves to reinforce the power of the researcher relative to that of the people whose lives are being studied. She challenges researchers to write in a language that does not alienate and exclude those who took part in the research, and to return information to the participants in the language in which it originated.

This prompts consideration of the purpose of research, and how the knowledge that has been jointly created by the researcher and participants is to be used. We must be honest about whether the real purpose is to further our own careers, to enhance the profiles of our various professions and thereby to reaffirm inequalities of power and access to knowledge;

or whether, through thinking about how we write, how we represent the voices of the participants in our research, and where we choose to present this information, we challenge and contest inequality and hierarchies of knowledge and make our research accessible to those of whom we write.

Shakespeare (1996) has highlighted the tendency for researchers to publish in those academic forums that will further their own careers, rather than enabling disabled people access to their findings. Thus, Oliver (1992) advocates a change in the social relations of research, with jointly constructed knowledge placed at the disposal of the researched as well as the researchers. He alludes to the 'inescapable fact' that, as researchers, 'we are the main beneficiaries of our own research activities' (Oliver 1997, p. 27).

Creating change

Shakespeare (1996) suggests that publishing research findings in an accessible language and in publications that are read by disabled people ensures that these people have access to information that *they* can use to influence policy and attain more control over their lives. My own study demonstrated how successful disabled people can be in this endeavour.

British Columbia, where my study was undertaken, is almost unique in Canada in enacting social policies that enable people with high spinal cord injuries to live autonomous lives in the community, where they have married, bought homes, raised children, enjoyed gainful employment and where they are enabled to employ their own staff to maintain the unremitting personal assistance they require. The history of deinstitutionalization for people with high tetraplegia in British Columbia began with some of the participants in my study, and although various professionals, politicians and policy makers have since allied themselves with this venture, it is important to recognize that the vision and momentum came from the institutionalized people themselves. That discharge from the rehabilitation centre to the community is now the norm, such that newly injured people with high tetraplegia in British Columbia are no longer sent to institutions (unless they so choose), suggests that these few pioneers have created a new 'norm' that has permeated not only the ideology of the medical professions, but through every level of government in British Columbia.

In light of the reality that the impetus for social changes that benefit disabled people tends, almost without exception, to originate with disabled people themselves (rather than from able-bodied researchers, clinicians, theorists or policy makers), I made a commitment to the study participants to publish my research findings in formats accessible to those who are most likely to make use of the information: disabled people. Thus, my first papers stemming from the research will be submitted to publications produced by and for disabled people, and suggested by the participants in my study. However, because the need to challenge and change societal attitudes was a central research finding (and specifically the pessimistic attitudes of health-care professionals), I shall also submit papers to various medical and therapy journals.

FURTHER REFLECTIONS

It has been observed that in speaking and writing about others 'I am engaging in the act of representing the other's needs, goals, situation, and in fact, *who they are*' (Alcoff 1991, p. 9). This is a daunting responsibility.

In writing about my attempts to involve members of the study population at every stage of the research planning, data collection, analysis and eventual dissemination of findings, it is difficult to avoid sounding self-satisfied; I am not. On the contrary, I am only too acutely aware that the politics of universities (including ethics committees), the requirements for the completion of an academic degree and the time constraints upon study participants all militate against the objective of maintaining a truly collaborative research partnership. None the

less, I believe that in continually striving to keep people and politics at the centre of our research endeavours we must continually reflect upon issues of power, appropriation and respect. We need to ask ourselves who we most wish to value our research (and to be honest about the implications of the answer).

QUALITY IN LIFE FOLLOWING HIGH SPINAL CORD INJURY

Following the onset of his own tetraplegia, Murphy (1987) pondered: 'Would one really be better off dead? ... [That] is the big question, for to answer it we will also have to ask what constitutes living' (p. 6). The reports of the participants in this study suggested that they did not feel they would be better off dead; indeed, several reported lives that are more focused, less superficial, more meaningful and more rewarding than before the injury. Their narratives suggest that since there is no culturally accepted script for how one should live witha high spinal cord injury, each individual had the unique opportunity to define their own possibilities. The daily life experiences of the participants therefore ranged between those who expressed great satisfaction in being employed, attending university or lecturing, and those whose primary occupation (and source of profound satisfaction) comprised watching their children, visiting family members or reading.

It was interesting to note that few, if any, of the dimensions that they deemed to be important contributors to the quality of their lives (e.g. attaining autonomy, deinstitutionalization, enjoying the 'taken for granted': relationships, sunshine, nature, a shower, being alone) would be included in standard quality of life measures.

From the results of this study I contend that there are no universal, objective or predetermined, measurable criteria for quality *of* life but that each individual will define their own interpretation of the quality *in* life, and that this may change over time and in response to changing circumstances.

CONCLUSION

The purpose of the research was to understand what kind of life is *possible* with a high spinal cord injury. It is my hope that by documenting these possible lives I may help to suggest alternative patterns for living for newly injured people, and contribute to facilitating this process by confirming the need for changes in social policy that support the philosophy of human rights for all disabled people. Future research should examine what kind of life is *typical* following such an injury, documenting the experience of institutionalization and consequent marginalization that is the more common scenario for people with these injuries.

The purpose of the chapter was to challenge researchers to be reflective, not solely about their social and personal positioning, but to examine the ways in which their philosophical and political orientation affects the social relations of research and hence accountability to their study participants. Irrespective of the chosen research methodology, every researcher is confronted with choices that relate to the balance of power between themselves and their study participants: choices that relate to every stage of the research process and subsequent dissemination of findings.

I have proposed that disability researchers should ask themselves:

- What are the purposes and objectives of the research?
- Who is likely to benefit from it?
- In what ways will disabled people participate in the research process?
- Who do we want to value our research?
- Does the research process reflect this?
- Will the research findings be published in formats accessible to those who are most likely to benefit from the information?

The degree to which power and knowledge are shared with the research participants will be influenced by the answers to these questions.

Acknowledgements

I am greatly indebted to the 15 people with high lesion tetraplegia, their families and assistants, who welcomed both me and my study.

The research upon which this chapter is based was generously supported by the following: UBC Graduate Fellowship, Rick Hansen Man in Motion Foundation Studentship, Social Sciences and Humanities Research Council of Canada Doctoral Fellowship.

REFERENCES

Alcoff L 1991 The problem of speaking for others. Cultural Critique Winter: 5–31

Bogdan RC, Biklen SK 1998 Qualitative research for education. An introduction to theory and methods, 3rd edn. Allyn & Bacon, Boston

Bury M 1982 Chronic illness as biographical disruption. Sociology of Health and Illness 4(2):167–182

Edwards R, Ribbens J 1998 Living on the edges. Public knowledge, private lives, personal experience. In: Ribbens J, Edwards R (eds) Feminist dilemmas in qualitative research. Public knowledge and private lives. Sage, London, pp 1–23

Field PA, Morse JM 1985 Nursing research. The application of qualitative methods. Chapman & Hall, London

Gerhart KA, Koziol-McLain J, Lowenstein SR, Whiteneck GG 1994 Quality of life following spinal cord injury: knowledge and attitudes of emergency care providers. Annals of Emergency Medicine 23(4):801–812

Good BJ 1994 Medicine, rationality and experience. University of Cambridge Press, Cambridge

Harris A 1996 Responsibility and advocacy: representing young women. In: Wilkinson S, Kitzinger C (eds) Representing the other. Sage, London, pp 152–155

Marcus GE, Fischer MMJ 1986 Anthropology as cultural critique. An experimental moment in the human sciences. University of Chicago Press, Chicago

Moore M, Beazley S, Maelzer J 1998 Researching disability issues. Open University Press, Buckingham

Morse JM 1994 'Emerging from the data': the cognitive process of analysis in qualitative inquiry. In: Morse J (ed) Critical issues in qualitative research methods. Sage, Thousand Oaks, CA, pp 23–43

Murphy RF 1987 The body silent. WW Norton, New York

Oliver M 1987 Re-defining disability: a challenge to research. Research, Policy and Planning 5:9–13

Oliver M 1992 Changing the social relations of research production? Disability, Handicap and Society 7(2):1–114

Oliver M 1997 Emancipatory research: realistic goal or impossible dream? In: Barnes C, Mercer G (eds) Doing disability research. Disability Press, Leeds, pp 15–31

Roy DJ 1992 Editorial: Measurement in the service of compassion. Journal of Palliative Care 8(3):3–4

Sandelowski M 1986 The problem of rigor in qualitative research. Advances in Nursing Science 8(3):27–37

Shakespeare T 1996 Rules of engagement: doing disability research. Disability and Society 11(1):115–119

Standing K 1998 Writing the voices of the less powerful. Research on lone mothers. In: Ribbens J, Edwards R (eds) Feminist dilemmas in qualitative research. Public knowledge and private lives. Sage, London, pp 186–202

Ward L, Flynn M 1994 What matters most: disability, research and empowerment. In: Rioux MH, Bach M (eds) Disability is not measles. New research paradigms in disability. L'Institut Roeher, North York, Ontario, pp 29–48

Zarb GJ, Oliver MJ, Silver JR 1990 Ageing with spinal cord injury: the right to a supportive environment? Thames Polytechnic and Spinal Injuries Association, London

FURTHER READING

Barnes C, Mercer G (eds) 1997 Doing disability research. Disability Press, Leeds

England K 1994 Getting personal: reflexivity, positionality and feminist research. Professional Geographer 46(1):80–89

Fuhrer MJ 1994 Subjective well-being: implications for medical rehabilitation outcomes and models of disablement. American Journal of Physical Medicine and Rehabilitation 73:358–364

Gluck SB, Patai D (eds) 1991 Women's words. The feminist practice of oral history. Routledge, New York

7

Exploring how rehabilitation students acquire cultural competency: methodology and ethical considerations

Sue Forwell

OVERVIEW

This chapter describes a longitudinal study that sought to explore how occupational therapy students understand a complex concept ('culture') through their academic curriculum and clinical fieldwork. The focus of the chapter concerns the inevitable power differential and inherent ethical issues in studies involving students and faculty, and the measures that were taken to address these important issues. The chapter will also explore confidentiality, participant recruitment, the involvement of research assistants and data analysis.

BACKGROUND TO THE STUDY

There has been little exploration in the professional literature of issues related to occupational therapy students' acquisition of cultural competency in the context of their preparation to become practising clinicians, although this is a required competency and one that should be more clearly understood. Thus, the impetus for the research discussed in this chapter was grounded in the concern that the preparation of future occupational therapists must address competency to practise in a multicultural society. The research was underpinned by such questions as: Do students have the skills and knowledge to address complex issues of multicultural practice? Did the students acquire knowledge of cross-cultural issues from their experience with the occupational therapy curriculum? What strategies do students use to manage cultural diversity in practice? Do students perceive themselves as competent for multicultural practice? These questions, suggested by numerous classroom discussions and from a variety of situations experienced during field-work, served to inform our perceived need to ensure a culturally sensitive occupational therapy curriculum at the University of British Columbia (UBC). In this chapter I will discuss the specific research methods that were chosen, and ethical issues that were considered or which emerged during the implementation of this 3-year longitudinal study.

The study (conducted in collaboration with Isabel Dyck) was designed to investigate students' perceptions of their skills, knowledge and attitudes necessary for cultural competency, and the educational experiences that shaped these factors. It was based on the premise that students require education that is attuned to contemporary social issues, including the sociocultural factors that influence a client's participation in therapeutic interventions. With this purpose in mind, and informed by the questions (outlined above) that motivated the study, the methods we chose (journal keeping and in-depth interviewing) were deemed appropriate to the research aims.

STUDY DESIGN

Recruitment

This study followed a cohort of students from entry to graduation in the 3-year occupational therapy programme at the School of Rehabilitation Sciences, UBC. Study participants were recruited from among newly admitted students to the programme. In order to respect the rights of the students to confidentiality and to protect them from real or perceived conflicts that might arise if the faculty members

conducted the face-to-face interactions during research, research assistants were involved in the project. These individuals were not members of the teaching faculty in the School of Rehabilitation Sciences.

Students were introduced to the research project by a research assistant during a class from which the instructor absented herself. The research assistant provided students with a written outline of the study, as well as a verbal description, and invited students to volunteer to participate by completing a form and returning it to her. Thus, only the research assistant knew which students had agreed to participate in the study.

Data collection

The methods of data collection used in this 3-year study were in-depth semi-structured interviews and journal keeping. Journal keeping (during the first and second years of fieldwork) was incorporated to provide students with a mechanism for recording situations they perceived to have cultural significance, as they occurred. The interviews were conducted to generate detailed descriptions of events outlined in the journals, and to ascertain students' reflections on various occurrences as they related to themselves, the profession of occupational therapy and, subsequently, their practice as therapists. These interviews occurred following the completion of annual school requirements, which allowed students to reflect on the whole year when considering the cultural experiences encountered during fieldwork.

Year 1

Data collection in the first year of the study began with the research assistant conducting baseline interviews with students in their own homes. During these interviews students were asked for various demographic details and their everyday life experiences with people of different cultural groups. They were also asked about any skills or attributes which they brought to the occupational therapy programme that they considered would be useful for practice, and their ideas about the skills and knowledge they would need (and anticipated learning) to be competent in working in a practice context of cultural diversity. These interviews occurred in the first few weeks of the school term in which students entered the programme. The baseline interviews were tape-recorded and then transcribed. The research assistant completed detailed field notes for each interview to provide context, offer an impression of the setting, describe her feelings about the interaction and the environment, and to explain problems or any disruptions that might have occurred (for more details of the study and analysis, see Dyck & Forwell 1997).

At the end of the first year of classroom studies, and before students began fieldwork, the research assistant provided each study participant with a journal, explaining its purpose and a suggested method for making entries. Students were asked to note cultural situations encountered during their fieldwork placements, commenting on what happened, the response to the situation, and their feeling or interpretation about the handling of the situation. No guidance was given concerning a preferred volume or frequency of entry(-ies), other than to note that entries were an individual decision. The journals served as a record of cultural incidents encountered during fieldwork placements, and triggered the students' memories of these incidents in their post-placement interviews with the research assistant. During placements the research assistant communicated with each student to respond to any uncertainties about maintaining the journals.

It is important to note that the students were not provided with definitions of 'culture', 'ethnicity' or 'race' by which they could interpret either culture or cultural situations. Our intention was to understand how the students perceived and understood these constructs, and how their interpretations changed over time. In this way we sought to avoid prescribing situations that we ourselves deemed to be of cultural significance. Thus, students responded

---

Box 7.1 Framework of questions asked in first post-placement interview

- ◆ Can you tell me about your first/recent clinical experience?
- ◆ Can you tell me about the client group you were working with, with reference to their ethnicity and sociocultural backgrounds? or What cultural groups were you working with?
- ◆ How did the content of the occupational therapy educational programme prepare you for such an experience?
- ◆ Can you comment on the integration of the classroom material into fieldwork? or What aspects of the classroom content were most significant?
- ◆ What further skills do you feel you need to develop in the future to work with people of different cultural backgrounds to yourself, or to manage subsequent cross-cultural situations?

---

to our research questions from their own understanding and perception of these constructs. Following the end of the first year of fieldwork the research assistant conducted the second interview to explore the students' experiences and their thoughts about the first-year curriculum. The discussions centred upon situations the students had experienced during fieldwork that had cultural meaning or impact for them, and what, if any, part of their classroom content had prepared them for these occurrences. These interviews were oriented to gain an understanding of students' perceptions of the ways in which their academic learning prepared them for fieldwork, and how their fieldwork experiences had assisted their learning about cultural differences. Box 7.1 shows the framework of questions asked during this post-placement interview. It should be noted that these questions were accompanied by probes that facilitated both a flow of information and accounts of student experiences. The research assistant kept detailed field notes of each interview.

Upon completing their placements many of the students no longer lived near the university; therefore, subsequent interviews were either arranged when they visited the area or were conducted on the telephone. The post-placement interviews ranged from 20 to 90 minutes and were tape-recorded and transcribed. The journals that were submitted to the research assistant were typed and the originals returned to the authors. To protect confidentiality, any text that identified either the student or the fieldwork site was removed from the transcribed interviews and typed journals.

Year 2

During the second year of the study, which included 8 months of classroom work followed by 3 months of fieldwork, the research assistant maintained contact with the study participants. The students received letters of appreciation for participating in year 1 of the project and a description of their proposed involvement for the second year. Prior to fieldwork, the research assistant again met with each study participant to provide journals similar to those used in the first year.

Once the students embarked on their fieldwork the research assistant corresponded with each participant to address questions or concerns relating to documentation in their journals.

Following 3 months of fieldwork, the second post-placement interviews were conducted. The

format of these interviews mirrored those that were completed at the end of the first year of the project, although the depth of questions was enhanced. Box 7.2 illustrates the framework of questions used in this post-placement interview.

The interviews were transcribed and journals typed with any identifying information removed (again the original was returned to the student). The research assistant continued to maintain a record of all contacts with the study participants, as well as detailed field notes of each interview.

Year 3

In the final year of data collection contact was again maintained between the research assistant and the study participants. Journals were no longer required during fieldwork in this year, because the focus of data collection was to obtain the students' perspectives and reflections on the past 3 years, and not exclusively on their final-year experiences. Post-placement interviews were conducted by the research assistant and were similar in format to those in the previous years. However, as the focus was on the past 3 years, the questions were somewhat different. Box 7.3 illustrates these questions. The

---

Box 7.2 Framework of questions asked in second post-placement interview

Clinical experiences
◆ Can you tell me about your most recent clinical fieldwork experiences, e.g. setting, population, cultural groups etc.?
◆ Can you tell me about some of the cultural issues that you encountered in your clinical fieldwork this year? Which experiences had the greatest impact on you?
◆ Was there a time when you felt that you handled a cultural issue particularly well, that you were particularly pleased with? What skills or strategies did you use?
◆ Was there a time when you felt uncomfortable dealing with a cultural issue? What skills or strategies did you use? Did you feel adequately prepared? (If 'no', what skills did you feel were lacking, or that you need to develop further?)

Status of efficacy beliefs
◆ We have talked about some of the cultural

issues that you have encountered this year: can you identify and describe some of the skills that you possess which enable you to deal effectively with cultural diversity in your work?
◆ How confident do you feel dealing with cultural diversity in your work, in general?

Impact of programme content
◆ Which parts of the curriculum, if any, have helped prepare you to deal with cultural diversity in your clinical fieldwork? Which aspects of the programme were the most significant?
◆ Which areas, if any, do you believe you will need to develop further to enhance your cultural competency?

Other
◆ Is there anything that I have missed that you would like to add or comment on?

Box 7.3 Framework of questions asked in third post-placement interview

◆ Can you tell me about your clinical fieldwork experiences, e.g. setting, population, cultural groups etc. over the past 3 years?
◆ How well prepared do you feel you are to work in settings in which there are many different cultural groups present?
◆ What, if anything, has helped to prepare you to work with people from other cultures:
  – in terms of content of courses?
  – in terms of process, i.e. sequencing of courses, role models, teaching methods?
  – in terms of fieldwork: considering both useful and detrimental experiences?
◆ What in your life outside of university, in the past 3 years, has helped prepare you to work with people from other cultures?
◆ What more do you think you might need to learn or what skills would you like to develop to enhance your ability to work effectively with people from other cultures?
◆ What resources or strategies would you use to improve your skills?
◆ In what ways do you think the occupational therapy programme could be improved?
◆ What are your thoughts on the possibility of any conflict between the fundamental core, or founding concepts of OT and working with culturally different clients?

---

interviews were again tape-recorded and then transcribed, with all information that might enable identification of the students, fieldwork sites or personnel removed.

PARTICIPANT PROFILE

There were 35 students in the class, of whom 19 initially volunteered to participate in the study; 17 completed the first year. Analysis of the initial interviews suggested a mature, culturally aware group, most of whom recounted a variety of experiences with people of different cultural backgrounds, reflecting the experience of living in a multicultural society. Students clearly drew upon these personal experiences in the interviews, with 15 participants highlighting 'cultural situations' occurring with or among their families. Of these, seven reported that at least one of their parents had immigrated to Canada.

Fourteen students reported experiences with other cultural groups while growing up. These occurred as a result of living in a community or attending a school that had a mix of cultural groups (of which the most commonly reported were First Nations and people of Chinese heritage). Twelve students reported extensive travel experience, among whom seven had been to Europe and two to Asia-Pacific Rim countries. Through volunteer and/or paid work 13 students reported a rich array of cultural experiences. While at university or college 11 students noted involvement in extracurricular activities, having a classmate, and/or taking a course that provided them with further cultural awareness.

This cohort of students had a vast array of cultural experiences and were familiar with culturally diverse situations. However, as a group they had limited experience with cultural diversity in the professional milieu, and minimal, if any, exposure to a theoretical framework to consider cultural issues.

DATA ANALYSIS

We reviewed the initial interview transcripts for emerging themes concerning students' experiences with other cultural groups. The research assistant provided summaries of each student's accounts and extracted demographic data. This analysis and aggregation of demographic data provided contextual information for the students' reflections of their fieldwork experiences. Through a systematic analysis, the researchers and assistants worked together, discussing initial 'hunches' about the data and coding procedures, arriving at a consensus on the themes that we felt arose from the data. The combination of systematic record keeping, different data sources and team analysis ensured the rigour and 'credibility' of the research (Denzin & Lincoln 1994) (this is discussed further in Chapter 10).

Our analysis of the post-placement interviews began with a review of a few transcripts, which enabled us to gain an overall sense of the data and to note initial thoughts about common issues and concepts. A systematic coding of transcripts led to the development of a number of categories, which were subsequently collapsed into initial themes through a process of continual comparison of the transcripts. We reached a consensus on the meaning of each of the emerging themes and the 'name' to be given to each of these. However, it was found that although some themes remained constant during analysis, others shifted and were open to various interpretations. This became somewhat problematic, particularly owing to the disaggregation of data and decontextualization that accompanies this method of analysis, particularly in light of the researchers' self-imposed distance from the data collection process (Atkinson 1992).

We subsequently employed a second strategy which preserved a greater sense of context, in which meanings were constructed by the students in the words and stories that they had chosen to relate. This strategy consisted of coding by 'story', each of which was one complete event as described by a student. The predominant theme drawn from each story then provided the core for comparison with other stories. This approach maintained the context of the evolving themes while continuing to build by enabling comparison between transcripts. In essence, this allowed the small coded units gleaned in the first strategy for analysis to be viewed in the larger context of situation as described by the students. In this way, themes emerging from the comparative method could be analysed while retaining the particularity and complexity of the contexts within which meanings were embedded. The journal entries were coded in a similar way and compared with the transcripts.

The analysis was made more complex because the students reported their experiences in different ways, and included description of clients' and staff responses to situations as well as their own. This had not been anticipated. Unlike many research studies, which involve talking to people about their experiences retrospectively, students in this study were asked to participate actively in creating the parameters of the study through their selection of the fieldwork situations they elected to describe. In this way there was, perhaps, a clearer interweaving of investigator–participant roles in creating knowledge, with the students acting in a more explicit co-researcher role than is usual.

HIGHLIGHTS OF FINDINGS

Hundreds of pages of data were collected in each of the 3 years of this research. Here the dominant themes that emerged are briefly outlined.

One was defined as 'Canadian-ness', wherein students implicitly or explicitly described their own cultural experiences within the context of their notion of mainstream Canadian culture. In another theme, labelled 'making sense of difference', students expressed their rationale for defining situations as being due to cultural influences, rather than to other possible explanations. (These two themes, 'Canadian-ness' and 'making sense of difference', are described in more depth in Dyck & Forwell 1997).

Other themes that were apparent in our data concerned professional issues relating to assessment or intervention, and to the potential tension between the ideals of client-centredness and those of independence.

Communication was another area in which students discovered challenges, particularly in the presence of language difficulties. Other groupings of themes related to social issues and included racism, issues of gender and issues relating to the family and caregiving.

These themes briefly highlight the issues to which our data have given voice. The complexity and richness of the data have served to challenge our thoughts and ideals about the cultural curriculum provided to our students.

ISSUES SPECIFIC TO THIS STUDY

A combination of issues, unique to the design and implementation of this study, necessitated careful initial planning and appropriate ongoing responses. Of these, six are outlined here, including recruitment and ethnic representation, confidentiality, power differentials between ourselves (as both faculty members and the researchers) and the student participants, 'distance' from the data, the role of the research assistant, and data sources.

Recruitment and ethnic representation

When students were asked about their own cultural identities all 17 stated that they were Canadian, although 12 indicated an additional cultural identity (one was Chinese and the rest declared a European ancestry). In total, 16 of the 17 students were white, approximately 95% of the participant pool. This did not reflect the composition of the class of 35 students, among whom there were two Indo-Canadians (5% of the class), six Asian-Canadians (18%) and 27 whites (77%). Although 23% of the class were of non-European ancestry, only one of these participated in the study; non-white students were therefore not proportionately represented among the study participants.

The students who participated in the study expressed a desire to reflect on the development of their cultural competency. The reason why the other 18 students in the class did not volunteer is not known, and we could only entertain hypotheses as to why they chose not to volunteer, such as a lack of time, a view that either the study was not relevant or the subject matter was not valuable, that the topic was not important or too threatening, and/or that the initial presentation by the research assistant was not well received. Three additional reasons might also be considered. First, perhaps the recruitment strategy might have served to attract white students, or was somehow viewed as a deterrent to non-white students. It is possible that because the research assistant who initially introduced the project was white – and despite conscious efforts to be inclusive – the initial introduction might have been perceived as unappealing to non-white students. Secondly, perhaps the fact that the investigators and members of faculty in the School of Rehabilitation Sciences were white was perceived to be a greater threat to non-white students, in that they were less trusting of the process structured to secure their anonymity. Thirdly, perhaps the topic of culture is something that, in the Canadian context, non-white students choose not to focus on. It is possible that for non-white students, participation in a study that attends to cultural difference might be viewed as undesirable in the light of their potential efforts to integrate into Canadian culture. Although there are likely to be several other possible reasons for this under-representation, it is valuable to consider these possible factors in selecting and structuring the methods for recruiting study participants in any future studies.

Alternative recruitment means had been considered: one was to randomly select students to participate based on a visible cultural mix. However, it was decided not to proceed in this way as we wished participation to be voluntary, and there were theoretical and ethical problems in singling out students on the basis of colour. Nonetheless, it could be argued that a personal invitation to potential participants might have increased interest, or promoted the perception that their input was of particular value. Another potential recruitment strategy that we had discussed was to introduce the project solely by providing written information, rather than having a verbal presentation as well, but the inclusion of the presentation was deemed important to allow potential participants to ask questions immediately and receive feedback, or to have concerns dealt with quickly. Another option would have been to have a second research assistant who was from a visible minority group to participate in the initial presentation. This would have provided students with a second person with whom they might have been able to identify.

Although several recruiting methods had been considered, we recognized that each had its own set of limitations. As investigators, we weighed the pros and cons of each method and argued for, and ultimately decided upon, the process that was eventually used.

Confidentiality

Ethical considerations were central to the integrity of the study and it was imperative that we addressed these issues, particularly given the context in which the study was conducted: a small class size, few faculty in the UBC Occupational Therapy Division, and the majority of fieldwork sites being located in a small geographical area. Under these circumstances normal engagement in the academic programme naturally led to familiarity between students, faculty and fieldwork educators at the fieldwork sites. As a result, a number of measures were necessary to assure students that their anonymity would be protected; to uphold the confidentiality of the clients, fieldwork educators and other fieldwork site personnel; and to ensure that the reputation of fieldwork sites was not compromised.

From the start of the study systematic and confidential record keeping, as well as consistent data management, were adopted. To protect their anonymity, students selected their own pseudonyms and these were used throughout the 3 years of the study. To avoid the possibility of recognizing the voices of participants, the researchers did not listen to the taped interviews: either the research assistant who had conducted the interview or the transcriber (who was otherwise uninvolved in the study) listened to and transcribed all the interviews. Journal entries were also typed to avoid the possibility that the researchers might recognize handwriting. Further, the research assistant removed all identifiers (such as the names of fieldwork setting, place names and names of people) from the interviews, journals and field notes, and replaced these with descriptions. This last procedure also served to protect the confidentiality of the fieldwork sites.

We did not read the signed consent forms completed by student participants, or the letters written to the students by the research assistant. These (and all other contact information about the students) were maintained by the research assistant.

It was our intention that, by paying close attention to these issues, students would be assured of their anonymity and feel more unencumbered to discuss the details of their experiences during fieldwork. The fieldwork educators and others with whom students worked at the fieldwork site also remained anonymous. Clients' identities were unknown, and so the study did not compromise their care.

Inherent power differential between investigators and study participants

As the primary investigators in this study, we are faculty members at the University of British Columbia and teach the student participants who volunteered for the study. It was therefore imperative that we recognize the real or implied unequal power relationships that exist between us and the student participants. This raises the issue of conflict of interest and is potentially contradictory to the intimate and open exchange and disclosure that is considered central to qualitative interviewing (Fontana & Frey 1994, Hammersley & Atkinson 1995). Further, '… special care should be taken to ensure that consent is freely given where subjects are in a subordinate position to the researcher … [and] the design of the research [should] minimize the risk of harm to the subject …' (Dickens 1979, pp. 2–3).

As a result, we structured the data collection process to minimize the inevitable power imbalance as much as possible by hiring a research assistant. Selection of this person was critical to the project because she was the only point of contact with students throughout the 3-year study. At no time during the 3 years were we in direct contact with study participants, nor did (do) we know which specific students were involved in the project.

'Distance' from the data

Although incorporating a research assistant into the study design did, in part, address issues related to the relationship between ourselves (as the investigators) and the student participants, this approach has its limitations. The primary one was the distance created between us, as researchers, and the data collection process and study participants. To reduce this shortcoming as much as possible, a number of strategies were adopted. Frequent meetings were held with the research assistant, particularly at the beginning of each new phase of the study, so that we could discuss the purposes of the interviews and journals and clarify any queries or concerns raised by either the assistant or the students. Following the interviews, we also held debriefing sessions with the research assistant. As well as maintaining detailed field notes of each interview, the research assistant also reported the step-by-step process of the study, including difficulties, as well as routine, non-problematic procedures.

Role of the research assistant

The role of the research assistant in this study was complex and required diverse skills. The assistant who was hired had demonstrated skills in interviewing and a knowledge of qualitative research methods, although she was unfamiliar with either rehabilitation or occupational therapy. She was responsible for the logistics and implementation of the initial recruitment of study participants and all ongoing contact with students, conducting the interviews and collecting journals.

The research assistant was the only contact with students. As a result, she liaised between students and ourselves to address issues that arose prior to and during data collection. It was necessary that the research assistant was sensitive to students' concerns regarding their need for confidentiality and their desire to articulate their experiences in a meaningful, reflective way. These were very important attributes that had an effect on the interview exchange and the data collected.

The research assistant also worked closely with us to contribute to the ongoing data analysis. Each year, after interviews were completed, the research assistant met with us to discuss the data collection process for that year and to embark on the initial stages of data analysis. As well as interfacing with students and ourselves, the research assistant was responsible for maintaining field notes, descriptions of methodological issues, copies of letters and consents, and records of all contacts with students. In addition to these she managed the data on the interview tapes and also the multiple copies of the transcribed interviews and journal entries. Unfortunately, we were unable to achieve our desired degree of continuity during the study, owing to the departure of our original research assistant and the consequent need to recruit another. This inevitably disrupted any rapport and trust that had been established between the students and the research assistant, and reduced the possibility of a consistent approach to interviewing and data collection.

Data sources

The use of more than one data source is believed to enhance the credibility of qualitative research (see Chapter 10). Of interest in this study are the types of data sources and the frequency of data collection. By using both interviews and journals, students were able to reflect on cultural situations that they identified during fieldwork, both privately (through journal entries) and with someone else (during the interview). These two formats also provided students with the opportunity to report both in writing and verbally. It was our hope that by using a mix of private, written reflection and discussion with the research assistant, we would not only gain a richness of data but accommodate the individual students' preferences for style of communication. The journals were designed to provide an immediate forum for reflection and documentation, in addition to providing a stimulus for further discussion with the research assistant in the context of the interviews.

The frequency of data collection allowed participants to reflect on their experiences and learning on several occasions, and to develop and build on those reflections over time. There were a total of four interviews and two periods of journal keeping during the 3 years of the study. Participants indicated that as a result of their involvement in this study – which required a recounting of situations they felt had cultural significance that occurred during fieldwork – they became more reflective and culturally aware. As one of the student participants said, 'The research itself was probably a good teaching tool ... because it helped us reflect ... helped in reflection and learning'. It was interesting to observe that there were no discrepancies between the accounts of cultural experiences described in the interviews and those reported in the journals, although some students recorded incidents in their journals that were not covered in the interviews. In most cases the data sources complemented and supplemented each other, providing richly textured descriptions of fieldwork experiences.

CONCLUSION

This chapter details the research methods and the specific methodological issues that arose in our 3-year study designed to explore the many aspects of how occupational therapy students perceive their skills, knowledge and attitudes for culturally competent practice. In designing the study we had paid careful attention to the research methods, including the strategy used to recruit student participants and the structure and process of data collection, which included semi-structured interviews and journal keeping.

The demographic profile of the study cohort showed that the majority of students were between 21 and 23 years old, Canadian-born single females, with 3 years' university education. Their collective cultural experiences prior to entering the occupational therapy programme were diverse and arose from multiple sources, including their families, travel, voluntary and/or paid work, and school experiences. A number of complex and sensitive issues and themes emerged from the data analysis, and have the potential to inform our occupational therapy education programme.

The methodological issues specific to this study related to ethnic representation of study participants (or, in this study under-representation), confidentiality of students and people at fieldwork sites, the inherent power differential in our position as faculty/researchers and our students as the study cohort, the pivotal role of the research assistant and the use of multiple data sources.

Considerable attention was given to these issues during the initial study design and continued throughout the data collection and analysis period. We continued to re-evaluate and respond to changing situations and concerns raised by students, non-participants and the research assistant throughout the research process. The approach chosen for this study and the emerging issues that related to the research design demonstrated the dynamic relationship between our research questions and the ethical parameters of the study itself.

Acknowledgements

Sandy Michener and Judy Bushnell were the two research assistants, whose input contributed greatly to the success of this study.

Funding for this research was provided through a grant from the British Columbia Health Research Foundation.

REFERENCES

Atkinson P 1992 The ethnography of a medical setting: reading, writing and rhetoric. Qualitative Health Research 2:453–457
Denzin NK, Lincoln YS 1994 Introduction: Entering the field of qualitative research. In: Denzin NK, Lincoln YS (eds) Handbook of qualitative research. Sage, Thousand Oaks, pp 1–17
Dickens BM (ed) 1979 Guidelines on the use of human subjects. Office of the Research Administration, University of Toronto
Dyck I, Forwell S 1997 Occupational therapy students' first year fieldwork experiences: discovering the complexity of culture. Canadian Journal of Occupational Therapy 64(7):185–196
Fontana A, Frey JH 1994 Interviewing: the art of science. In: Denzin N, Lincoln Y (eds) Handbook of qualitative research. Sage, Thousand Oaks, pp 361–376
Hammersley M, Atkinson P 1995 Ethnography: principles in practice, 2nd edn. Routledge, London

FURTHER READING

Hammersley M, Atkinson P 1995 Ethnography: principles in practice, 2nd edn. Routledge, London

Holstein JA, Gubrium JF 1994 Phenomenology, ethnomethodology, and interpretive practice. In: Denzin NK, Lincoln YS (eds) Handbook of qualitative research. Sage, Thousand Oaks, pp 262–272

Patton MQ 1990 Qualitative evaluation and research methods. Sage, Newbury Park, CA

8

Working with theory in qualitative research: an example from a study of women with chronic illness (multiple sclerosis)

Isabel Dyck

KEY POINTS

interpreting data; interview narratives; feminist theory; women and the paid workplace; body and identity; multiple sclerosis

CHAPTER CONTENTS

OVERVIEW

The issue of theory in qualitative research is approached from different perspectives, but common to all is the premise that analyses are inductive and concept generating, rather than deductive and hypothesis testing. That is, interpretations are grounded in the data generated from the research; it is from such narrative data, whether in the form of field notes, interview transcripts, videos, photographs, media text, documents or other forms of non-numerical data, that ways of understanding the topic at hand are generated. Often, as in research based primarily on the in-depth interview, conceptualizations rely heavily on the voices of those with whom we conduct research. Their experiences are commonly viewed as the primary data, together with field notes describing the contextual features of an interview and its 'subject', from which categories and conceptualizations are generated. How we conceptualize the experiences of research participants, as expressed in the narratives that are co-constructed between them and the researcher, however, is informed by the researcher's insights and 'hunches' which in turn are informed by existing interpretive concepts from the literature and the researcher's social positioning. It is this latter idea that is most troubling for the new qualitative researcher, particularly if previously educated in the positivist paradigm of the natural sciences and quantitative method, where 'objectivity' and personal distance from the data are viewed as imperative.

This chapter aims to address the issue of working with theory in the interpretation of qualitative data. It is based on the notion that researchers cannot enter a study with a blank mind, open to unmediated 'pure' data. Even if they are unaware of theoretical orientation, their very choice of research topic and research design is necessarily framed by a perspective laden with ideas and concepts coming from a particular academic discipline or professional body of knowledge, as well as personal experiences. This is not to suggest that qualitative research is therefore 'subjective' in a sense that in some way invalidates the findings of a study, but rather to argue that empirical research and theory may be closely intertwined. Yet how theory informs a study varies. Some studies are more descriptive than others, telling a detailed story about the situation and people that are of central interest to the researcher. Other studies work more consciously with theoretical issues, challenging and refining existing concepts or developing new ways of understanding a topic. This chapter focuses on how theory and interpretation of qualitative data may be consciously intertwined when the aim of the research is not confined to description, but is interested in theoretical concerns. Ongoing theoretical development is dependent on closely argued and nuanced analysis grounded in data, just as the interpretation of data may be informed by the sensitizing concepts of theory. That is, concepts from existing theories colour the lenses through which the researcher reads study data, informing interpretation in a way that allows them to confirm, refine or contest existing conceptualizations. Such a working *with* theory (as opposed to imposing theory, which suggests forcing data into predetermined categories) can take us beyond description of experience to a greater understanding of the many dimensions of complex social phenomena such as disability.

I discuss how ideas from social theory, particularly that developed in feminist scholarship, helped me in the analysis of women's workplace experiences following a diagnosis of multiple sclerosis (MS). One area of concern, pervading many academic disciplines influenced by the intellectual 'turn' of postmodernism, is that of 'difference' and identity, and how these are embodied at particular historical junctures (see Fox 1993 for its use in interpreting health issues). This includes an interest in how identities are constituted and have the potential to be transformed in connection with axes of difference, such as gender, class, 'race', sexual orientation or disability. Ultimately this direction in scholarship is concerned with issues of diversity in society, including issues of social justice pertaining to the identification of people as 'different'. In the field of disability studies, and of relevance to occupational therapy, there is a focus on understanding the construction of 'disabled' identities, whether in perception of self or as imposed as social identities by others.

In my own research I have been interested in the social and spatial processes involved in such identity formation, and the social consequences of such identification. In asking these questions I am informed by theoretical perspectives which recognize that meanings about the body and disability are constructed within sets of social relations and spatial structures that are specific to time, place and culture. The data of the study discussed in this chapter could have been analysed in a different way, but this is a theoretical area I see as contributing to our understanding of the complex interconnections between the individual and their environment, currently of interest in developing the conceptual base of occupational therapy. At the same time, it is important to note that the issue of identity, which is the main topic of this chapter, was not imposed on the data because of the author's interests: rather, it emerged as a primary concern for the women participating in the study as they talked about their experiences in the workplace following diagnosis with MS.

The purpose of this chapter is, first, to show how working with theoretical ideas in the interpretation of qualitative data can enhance our understanding of the complex relationships between the individual and society that shape people's experiences of chronic illness and the meaning of disability; and secondly, to indicate how this type of knowledge can be translated into the conceptual development of occupational therapy. In this chapter I briefly outline general theoretical ideas pertinent to the analysis of narrative accounts that constitute the main data of qualitative studies. I go on to describe briefly how analysis proceeded in the study of data (see also Chapter 2) and identify the main issues described by the women participating in the study in connection with their struggles in the paid workplace. Following this, I discuss how particular theoretical ideas informed this analysis, and conclude with a commentary on how such theoretically informed interpretation can contribute to occupational therapy's knowledge base. The focus here is to discuss how theory informed the analysis (a more detailed explanation of the qualitative analysis can be found in Dyck 1995, 1996, 1998, 1999).

CONSTRUCTING KNOWLEDGE AND THE INTERPRETATION OF QUALITATIVE DATA

Feminist scholars have been particularly influential in deconstructing what we tend to accept as taken-for-granted knowledge; that is, they have shown that all knowledge is developed within particular contexts, both historical and cultural. In the past knowledge was primarily constructed from viewpoints grounded in male experiences, as men tended to occupy the positions of greater power in creating knowledge, whether as academics or otherwise, with which we understand and explain our worlds. Haraway (1988), a noted biologist and feminist scholar, suggests that the very notion of 'objectivity' is open to question, as all knowledge comes from a view from 'somewhere' and therefore is partial and incomplete. We are not, as the scientific paradigm would suggest, able to have universal knowledge that gives us a total picture of a phenomenon. There is no singular truth. Beer (1997) talks eloquently of qualitative research in terms of obtaining 'a certain slant of light' on subject participants' lives; we are, through careful and thoughtful investigation, permitted a view from their 'somewhere' that may be new to us, as researchers with different experiences. That is, of course, a central aim of qualitative research: we aim to understand another's experience from their perspective.

Gaining this different slant of light does not necessarily stop at representing those experiences: we may be interested in trying to discover those relationships and structures in society which create that 'different experience' with which we were not previously familiar. Furthermore, there is a questioning of whether narratives gained through interviews can represent 'pure experience', as they need to be understood as joint constructions of study participants and researcher. Certainly, in-depth interviews produce many pages of transcription, full of detail about the lives of those we interview, and necessarily we report in a somewhat selective way on what emerges from the data. Strong themes across transcripts catch our attention as being worthy of further exploration.

A strong theme of the study discussed here was that of disclosure: to whom, when and in what situations was this an issue for women? We found that the paid workplace was a space particularly problematic for women in their decision to disclose or not. Identity and income issues were of particular concern. It was in interpreting the data about these issues that I found that theoretical insights from post-structural feminism, social theory about the body and geographical work on identity helped to locate the women's individual experiences in wider social and spatial relations and distributions of power. That is, it helped to draw out some of the complex interconnections between the individual and different dimensions of environment. But before going on to the specifics of working with these theoretical ideas in the analysis, I describe a little about the study, the analysis and the themes emerging from the women's narrative accounts. This mirrors the actual study process.

THE STUDY: WORKING WITH THE INTERVIEW NARRATIVES AND THE INTERPRETIVE ACT

The study was informed in a general way by a sociopolitical model of disability, which is consistent with approaches that understand disability as a social construct (Jongbloed & Crichton 1990, Oliver 1990). That is, the meaning and experience of impairments will be shaped by social relations, spatial structures and discourses about health, illness and disability. All these will be specific to time, place and culture, and they will shape the resources made available to people who have impairments or chronic illness, and the conditions under which they live and work. This approach necessitates that we look at the interaction of the individual and society in order to fully understand the meanings and con-sequences of disease symptoms for people in particular phases. In order to do this the study used a mixed design (see Chapter 2) of in-depth interviewing followed by a questionnaire survey. Those 31 women who were employed and participated in the qualitative phase of the study are the focus in this chapter. They ranged in age from 25 to 49 years; 14 were married or in common-law relationships, and 17 were single, separated or divorced.

The interviews provided rich detail and textured accounts of the women's responses to the knowledge of their diagnosis, and the subsequent issues they faced in the home, their neighbourhoods, and in paid employment. Overall we had many pages of descriptions of how women responded to their illness and managed their changing abilities. The task of analysis began with a careful reading through of all the transcripts by both researchers. This involved initial categorization, followed by the two researchers comparing and contrasting the emerging themes, among which were two of specific importance to women in the paid workplace: those of uncertainty and identity,

particularly for those women who termed themselves 'invisible'. Most of the women had experienced a period of such hidden disability, in that although they might feel ill and be experiencing, for example, sensory, mobility and fatigue problems, they appeared healthy to others. It is a time when identity issues, and the associated dilemma of disclosure, become particularly acute for women, and their accounts described the various strategies they used in attempts to keep their diagnosis and limiting symptoms hidden.

EMERGING THEMES

Uncertainty

This theme embraced different types of uncertainty. There was medical uncertainty over the cause, course and prognosis of the disease, and the efficacy of methods of symptom management for a specific woman. The women expressed personal uncertainty in two main areas: that of the day-to-day experience of symptoms, which varied in severity and could be transient, and concerning their long-term ability to continue to perform as usual in terms of their identities as, for example, mothers, wives, lovers, workers and friends. For some this was complicated by advice from their physician; such advice varied widely, with some women being encouraged to continue as usual, whereas others came to doubt their ability to mother 'appropriately' or to work, following cautions from their physician. Furthermore, women found the language of biomedicine inadequate to describe dimensions of illness that were not purely physical, for example the uncertainties of day-to-day performance as they were cir-cumscribed and interpreted in the particular social contexts of home, neighbourhood and the paid workplace. This was further complicated for those who experienced contradictions between the diagnosis and their current feelings of illness or of being well. This became of particular issue for some women in the context of their paid workplace: for example, those with hidden disability – the 'invisibles' – might look well but in fact were struggling with various bodily changes which affected their ability to work, although inconsistently. This, it should be noted, was also an issue in the home concerning domestic labour for some women (Dyck 1998).

Struggling with identity

Women with invisible disabilities expressed concern over how disclosing that they had MS might affect the way they were considered and treated at work. Fear of discrimination was common. One woman who had disclosed felt she had been harassed out of her job as a retail clerk (shop assistant); others who had not disclosed were concerned that they might lose their job, or not be given promotion opportunities. Another concern for women seeking employment was that disclosure might lose them the chance of a job, or jeopardize their eligibility for disability insurance schemes. These issues were particularly salient for single women or others dependent on their own income for financial stability. Threats to an 'able' identity were voiced by several women as they talked of their employment experiences. This was a predominant theme in the narrative accounts. There were ambiguities for some women: on the one hand they were aware that their changing physical capacities relating to MS, such as fatigue, disturbances in coordination or sight, and difficulties in walking or standing for long periods of time, made some work tasks difficult; but on the other they felt they were still capable of working. Experiencing a 'destabilization' of an identity as 'able' was common.

The importance of an able identity in the context of the paid workplace for women is illustrated by the comment made by Deirdre, a single woman in her early 40s:

... we have this culture that if you don't have a job ... you're not a person. [And] then if you tell that you don't have a job because you're on long-term disability – I mean, you're even less of a person ... Even if you are only working [part-time] you have a place – you have an employer and you have a job and you have this thing that you do.

Later in the interview she talked of her job in terms of 'I'm ... not marginalized. I'm legitimate.' The idea of feeling 'legitimate' ran through many women's stories. Whereas for Deirdre feeling legitimate related to her position in the world as a person with a 'thing that you do', for others the idea of legitimacy also drew on discrepancies between what a woman felt she was able to do and what others might or did expect of her in light of a diagnosis of MS. Again this was frequently tied to identity concerns, as illustrated by the following:

It's up to me to say whether I'm being affected to the point that I cannot do my job, not for them to say that. So, I just don't feel that I should be sick at this point in my life. Because I'm not ready, you know?

One of my big tasks since I've been diagnosed has been trying to ... deal with changing [my] image ... I just don't want to identify with the disabled.

The struggle with threats to a previous able identity often involved an attempt to hide any difficulties women had with particular tasks at work, or the demands of the pace of work or a long day. Women who had not disclosed devised various ways of concealing symptoms from clients, co-workers or employers. In this way they were able to defer public knowledge of their diagnosis and the meanings attributed to it by others in the workplace. Some women could manage to work all day and recover at home, curtailing their social life to enable this recovery. When problems became obvious or limitations could not be dealt with easily, women sometimes attributed transient difficulties, such as stumbling or fatigue, to alternative problems, for example a sprained ankle, a bad back, or 'flu. These conditions were seen as less stigmatizing than a diagnosis of MS.

However, the ability of a woman to conceal performance difficulties was contextualized within specific workplaces and depended on a variety of factors, in addition to the actual tasks. They included, for example, her ability to order her tasks and day; the extent to which she worked alone or with others; the closeness of supervision; the physical settings within which her work took place; and specific workplace cultures that might emphasize a high performance or be less demanding of workers. As might be expected, those women most able to employ concealment strategies were those of higher seniority and/or in professional jobs where there was considerable leeway in how a woman could pace and organize her work. In the context of paid employment, MS therefore was experienced differently according to class positioning. Apart from women in professional positions, many workplaces, such as in retail, sales and other service occupations (where women's employment is concentrated), are structured in a way that is unforgiving of physical difficulties. Nevertheless, the anticipated stigma and possible discrimination as a result of revealing a diagnosis was experienced regardless of class.

The struggle to retain employment was complicated by the different ways in which the diagnosis could be used. The authority of a biomedical diagnosis and the tensions it produces in women's experiences is hinted at by the women in their narratives as they describe their dilemma concerning disclosure. On the one hand it legitimates their claims to illness, when others might doubt this – for example for women whose symptoms do not show; on the other hand it declares them to be diseased, in essence somehow suspect, with a body that is 'deviant'. Disclosure of the diagnosis has a double edge: this is something many women are aware of. They often realize that the diagnosis may be used in different ways as they negotiate their position in the labour force, as it does not convey one single meaning. It is the risk and uncertainty of how it may be 'read' that concerns women. Will colleagues and employers be supportive? Will they treat the woman differently? There is the risk of loss of employment, especially in the private sector, with the consequent loss of income and social marginalization. Yet the diagnosis can uphold a woman's disability status and gain her access to disability benefits and pensions. In a supportive work environment the diagnosis may result in help on the job or rearrangement of the physical environment, work tasks or hours to allow her to continue working.

These are risks a woman takes on declaring her diagnosis. Similarly, her identity becomes an issue: will her disease category dominate in the way people now treat her? In the workplace the strategies women adopted were in response to the varied concerns they had over the interpretation of the diagnosis and the meaning given to it in the particular context of the workplace. This was a particular concern where there was a disjuncture between what a woman felt, and felt able to accomplish at work, and a diagnosis that evokes meanings of disability. In their experience – often one of considerable uncertainty as to day-to-day symptoms – a diagnosis that might imply disability was problematic. Either way, disclosure of the diagnosis was, as one woman put it, like 'coming out'. The woman's knowledge of her diseased body becomes public knowledge, although the range of who is to be included in this 'public' will vary. The workplace is often the last arena in which disclosure is made, after family and friends. The woman's identity as 'able' is now open to interpretation and negotiation.

IDEAS FROM THEORY: INTERPRETING THE WOMEN'S ACCOUNTS

The rich accounts of the women's day-to-day experiences, concerns and management strategies are valuable in helping us understand the struggles the women had with the people, places and activities in their lives. Such descriptions give us an insight into the typical and sometimes unique concerns of study participants from their perspective – Beer's 'certain slant of light'. But what can we make of such descriptions in developing a body of knowledge concerned, for example, with theorizing the intersections between the individual and society (as a layering of environments). Here the act of interpretation, already in motion in the ways in which we select from the stories we are told and then construct written descriptions of them for our readers, draws more consciously on concepts from existing literature. The surprises common to qualitative research are not subdued by this process: rather, they become even more intriguing as one puzzles with them in analysis. Such working with data is a recursive process, data informing theory and theory informing the interpretation of data.

Every discipline and body of literature has core concerns, debates and arguments that are being investigated in the ongoing development of knowledge and refinement of concepts. As a social geographer working at the interface with the health sciences, and particularly occupational therapy, I come with various interests and interpretive 'aids' to analysis. From an occupational therapy perspective I am interested in what conceptual tools we can use to better understand the environment and its various dimensions in relation to occupational performance. As a geographer, with a collection of nuanced understandings of space and place and their relationship to human experience and action, I am interested in how these can aid understanding disability as a social phenomenon and personal experience. Given occupational therapy's central concern with appropriate ways to approach the 'differently abled' in clinical reasoning, which conceptualizes the client and their occupational performance as closely interconnected with various environmental components, there are several points of connection with current reflections in social theory. Work on 'difference', identity and the body, for example, has currency for occupational therapy research that aims to enhance understanding of disability and disability experience. Feminist theory brings a further dimension to these ideas, emphasizing the gendered character of experience.

Difference, identity, body

Although there is a broad consensus that gender does make a difference to experience, and in many situations women are a disadvantaged group – particularly those with impairments and chronic illness – it is also recognized that other axes of difference interweave with gender in forging experience. These include, for example, class, 'race', sexual orientation, age and citizenship. The close relation between difference,

identity and the body is an area currently being explored within this overall interest in the diversity of people's experiences in the world. Included in this exploration is how different spaces, such as homes, workplaces and various city spaces that have particular meanings about appropriate performance within them, mediate the experience of identity. Feminists and other scholars influenced by Foucault's work (see, for example, Foucault 1976, 1979) have been interested in how dominant ideas in society, such as those of science and medicine, exert considerable power in defining what is 'normal' and what is 'deviant'. Ways of defining difference may have profound implications on people's lives.

Those scholars who do not accept that people's experiences can be explained through unitary, homogeneous categories such as 'woman', 'disabled' or 'black', point to the fluidity of identity and its multifaceted quality, so that aspects of a person's identity may be more important in some contexts than others. For example, in some situations a woman's identity as a mother might be more salient than her identity as a paid worker, but her identity as a mother and as someone 'disabled' may become extremely important to how she is regarded by others in society. For example, she may be discouraged from having children and be thought not capable of raising a child in terms of cultural norms about 'good mothering'. Similarly, a person who is both disabled and black may face particular barriers in obtaining employment, and another person's access to benefits may depend on their categorization as 'disabled' by a classificatory system that takes inadequate account of that person's own knowledge and experience of their capacity to work. What is important here to note is that self-identification may not always match social categorization, whether informally in everyday social interaction or through systems of categorization that are backed by policy, authority of certain types of knowledge, or strongly held cultural norms. Similarly, to be identified in a particular way may lead to different social and personal experiences in different places and political economies.

To help understand these variations theoretically, literature that draws a close link between the body, 'difference' and identity has made a distinction between the corporeal body and the discursive body (see, for example, Shilling 1993, Grosz 1994). This thinking asks us to acknowledge a distinction between the biological, material body and a body that is 'inscribed' or 'marked' by powerful 'discourses' (or narratives circulating in society which interpret and describe the world) about such a body that have profound effects on a person's position in society and how he or she may use his or her physical capacities. For example, cultural norms about womanhood, appropriate mothering, family structure, femininity and masculinity pervade many aspects of everyday life, ordering the structure and organization of the labour market and social policy as well as shaping what are seen as appropriate activities for men and women to do in their everyday lives.

Similarly, ideas about what is 'different' from dominant cultural norms will shape the resources available to people in managing their lives, and how they are perceived. In the language of poststructuralism, which focuses on the notion of discourse, bodies – whether feminine, masculine, 'raced' or 'disabled' – are discursively produced or marked by dominant stories or scripts circulating in society about what men or women do, about disability, about what people of a certain phenotype and cultural background are like. It is against the normative ideas of dominant groups that 'others' (as opposed to those at the centre of a society, e.g. 'white', male, able-bodied) are discursively constructed. They are perceived to be (and made) different through a range of social practices that emphasize such distinctions, and which may be encoded in policy (Sasoon 1987, Pulkingham 1998).

So, where does this take us in the case of women diagnosed with MS and their employment issues? We can see them struggling with changes in their physical capacities – their material or corporeal bodies – and the considerable uncertainty in their day-to-day

ability to carry on as usual, together with the longer-term uncertainty that goes with the diagnosis of MS. They are also struggling with threats to their identities: both their self-identification as women and capable workers (and in their private lives as mothers, wives, lovers and friends) and their social identification as 'different', as 'other', as no longer able. Their 'performative acts', in the words of Butler (1990), no longer consistently uphold their identities as able, as feminine (in terms of culturally dominant norms and associations with the home), as important contributors to society through their work. Yet at times they remain capable workers, their impairments are invisible to those who monitor their workplace performance etc., and in some cases they are in remission or have benign disease with few, mild and transient symptoms. These latter women may, indeed, be without symptoms for long periods of time, but the diagnosis is there. They are 'marked' with the disease. Diagnosis, backed by the powerful authority of biomedical science and its practitioners, inscribes the body. It is itself a discourse (a cultural discourse rooted in Western scientific methods) about bodies, what has gone wrong with them, what can be expected from them, and, by implication, their capabilities and what resources, if any, should be made available in the light of the material body's changing capacities. Being inscribed or marked as 'other' in this way may have profound implications for their future lives, not just in terms of deteriorating physical capacities and feelings of illness (although this is not intended to discount these), but as their self- and social identities as being 'able' are eroded. Becoming 'disabled' formally and socially may close off employment opportunities, although it may also provide access to benefits designed for the 'disabled'. When translated into policy about access to disability income, there is a dichotomy drawn around the categories of 'able' or 'disabled', yet for most women this was not their experience. Policy does not have a category in between disabled or able which recognizes changing abilities from day to day or over time. Several women, in fact, did volunteer work when not able to match the regular hours and demands of the paid workforce.

The point here is that the material and the discursive bodies cannot be separated. It is not the case that a woman experiences one or the other, or that the experience of physical suffering is not given credence in theorizing which emphasizes the discursive construction of the body, but rather that they are closely intertwined. So closely intertwined, that the powerful discourse of biomedicine, which is itself a cultural construction (Good 1994), is taken for granted as the depiction with the most authenticity. Yet if we heed the women's accounts of their experiences, a focus solely on the material/corporeal body without consideration of the power of cultural inscriptions of 'other', we see examples of the authority of biomedicine mediating the women's experiences of their unpredictable, material bodies. As Wendell (1996, p. 122), suffering from chronic fatigue syndrome, states: '... my subjective descriptions of my bodily experience need the confirmation of medical descriptions to be accepted as accurate and truthful'. The diagnosis is a representation of the body of considerable authority that women accept or resist to different extents, according to their experiences and the context within which their diagnosis is being interpreted. Either way, their 'able self' is open to threat and renegotiation as they respond in various ways to the issues they encounter in their everyday life, including the workplace. Their workplace strategies are ones in which they represent themselves in a way that supports ableness as opposed to disablement, in opposition to a discourse of disease which may or may not match their own experiences of their corporeal or material body at a given time. As the women with MS in the study struggle with identity issues as they attempt to manage troublesome changes and failings of their material body, and to avoid disclosure, they are in effect delaying their public marking as 'different', as 'other'. They are resisting their representation as having deviant bodies and, with that, the doubt cast on their identities as 'whole' women.

CONCLUSION

The women in the study who are struggling with employment issues that focus on the material body and its capacities, are also struggling with identity issues and categorization as 'disabled' that will mediate ensuing life experiences. Some of these identity issues are at one level confined to their personal lives, but this personal life is also pervaded by a 'public' discourse of disease and disability, backed by biomedical science and policy entangled with this, that pervades social thought and understanding of 'disability'. Such a discourse intermingles with discourses about femininity and other axes of difference which all shape how impairments and illness are regarded, and what resources are seen as appropriate to provide. Although this study focuses on women in specific workplace environments in Canada and in a province with a particular structuring of benefits and available resources, women in other places may have different experiences, as the particularities of place – in both its social and its spatial organization – mediate how the body diagnosed with MS is experienced.

The interview narratives, in addition to Beer's 'slant of light', also provide insight into the interconnections between the individual and society, including the power relations permeating society's dominant discourses that define the 'normal' (whether concerning the body, health, ability or performance) and pervade the taken-for-granted dimensions of everyday life. Hence although the focus of such research is on the experiences of the study participants, it also provides an entry point from which to investigate the wider relations and discourses in society that pervade the experience of 'difference' – in this case the difference of disability. If aspects of society which are powerful in circumscribing the experience of disability are neglected in analysis, there is the danger of using a construct of disability which is potentially client-blaming through a focus on the individual as somehow separate from context. This is not to devalue empirical work which focuses primarily on description of the experiences of disability of different groups. This work clearly brings insight to the personal lives of those with disabilities of which we are otherwise unaware. But in working with social justice issues it is necessary to go beyond an individual: taking individual–environment interconnections seriously means working to understand wider social and spatial relationships that shape the meanings and management of the 'different body'. In doing this the researcher needs to engage with existing interpretations of such relationships and their influence on individual actions and experience.

For occupational therapists, using theory in interpretation in qualitative research means developing the theoretical 'arm' of the profession. How this is to be translated into practice is another step. It may not be direct. But as a beginning, having a wider understanding of the links between individual actions and society (including the dominant discourses that circulate and shape the organization of institutions, including health-care and disability policy) can aid clinical reasoning through analysis of the environmental influences on the occupational performance of clients. How we think about issues has potential influence on how we identify appropriate intervention. Interpretation of qualitative data with a conscious use of theory means not only describing the experiences of those we study, but also putting forth an interpretive position and entering debates about the adequacy of existing conceptualizations of the phenomena we are interested in and observe. For example, the study emphasizes that, just as we would expect clinical intervention to be one part of and an interruption in an ongoing narrative of a client (Mattingly 1991), we need to understand that such a personal narrative is also shaped and its course defined by powerful normative narratives, including that of the biomedical diagnosis, circulating in society that influence access to resources and opportunities for people suffering from chronic illness, such as MS, in a variety of ways as they inform social and disability policy. In effect we are placing the client more firmly within 'environment', tracing the complex interweaving of the interconnections between the two.

Acknowledgements

The study was funded by grants from the British Columbia Health Research Foundation and the Social Sciences and Humanities Council of Canada. Co-investigator was Lyn Jongbloed and the research assistant, who conducted many of the interviews, was Roberta Bagshaw.

REFERENCES

Beer D 1997 'There's a certain slant of light': the experience of discovery in qualitative interviewing. Occupational Therapy Journal of Research 17:110–129
Butler J 1990 Gender trouble: feminism and the subversion of identity. Routledge, New York
Dyck I 1995 Hidden geographies: the changing lifeworlds of women with multiple sclerosis. Social Science and Medicine 40:307–320
Dyck I 1996 Whose body? Whose voice? Atlantis 21:54–62
Dyck I 1998 Women with disabilities and everyday geographies. In: Kearns RA, Gesler WM (eds) Putting health into place: landscape, identity and well-being. Syracuse University Press, Syracuse, pp 102–119
Dyck I (1999) Body troubles; women, the workplace and negotiations of a disabled identity. In: Butler R, Parr H (eds) Mind and body spaces: geographies of disability, illness and impairment. Routledge, London (in press)
Foucault M 1976 The birth of the clinic. Tavistock, London
Foucault M 1979 Discipline and punish. Tavistock, London
Fox NJ 1993 Postmodernism, sociology and health. Open University Press, Buckingham
Good B 1994 Medicine, rationality and experience. Cambridge University Press, Cambridge
Grosz E 1994 Volatile bodies: towards a corporeal feminism. Indiana University Press, Bloomington
Haraway D 1988 Situated knowledges: the science question in feminism and the privilege of partial perspective. Feminist Studies 14:575–595
Jongbloed L, Crichton A 1990 A new definition of disability: implications for rehabilitation practice and social policy. Canadian Journal of Occupational Therapy 57:32–38
Mattingly C 1991 The narrative nature of clinical reasoning. American Journal of Occupational Therapy 45:998–1005
Oliver M 1990 The politics of disablement. Macmillan, London

Pulkingham J 1998 Remaking the social divisions of welfare: gender, 'dependency', and UI reform. Studies in Political Economy 56:7–48

Sasoon AS 1987 Women and the state. Hutchinson, London

Shilling C 1993 The body and social theory. Sage, London

Wendell S 1996 The rejected body. Routledge, London

FURTHER READING

Olesen V 1994 Feminisms and models of qualitative research. In: Denzin NK, Lincoln YS (eds) Handbook of qualitative research. Sage, Thousand Oaks, pp 158–174

Reinharz S 1992 Feminist methods in social research. Oxford University Press, Oxford

Understanding another life: using qualitative research in undergraduate education

Toby Wendland   Karen Hammell

OVERVIEW

This chapter is based on a paper written as part of an undergraduate rehabilitation science course as a method for a student to understand how an ethnographic interview can be used to gain new insight into another person's life. The focus is on demonstrating how an exercise in qualitative methods – specifically conducting and reflecting upon the process of an ethnographic interview – may be used as a tool for undergraduate students to understand the 'other' and thus inform a more reflective approach to practice.

The use of the ethnographic interview will be placed in its intellectual and philosophical context: contemporary moves within health care towards client-centred practice; and the interrelated need for qualitative methods of assessment to ensure that intervention is based upon a client-centred, rather than a therapist-centred, perspective of problems and concerns.

The chapter presents three voices. The first is that of Karen Hammell, who was a graduate teaching assistant for Dr Isabel Dyck's fourth-year occupational therapy class in qualitative research methods at the time when this student assignment was written. The second is that of 'Robert', and the third is that of Toby Wendland, who presented Robert's story, reflected upon his own place within the interview encounter and contemplated the impact of this interview upon his undergraduate education and subsequent professional practice.

INTRODUCTION

Fourth-year occupational therapy students at the School of Rehabilitation Sciences of the University of British Columbia undertake a 13-week course entitled 'An introduction to scientific inquiry', which is divided into two sections to address both quantitative and qualitative methodologies. Isabel Dyck, who presents the qualitative methodology section, explains that the purpose of this brief course is not to prepare students to conduct research, but rather to identify research problems amenable to a qualitative methodology, to demonstrate a knowledge of methods, research designs and types of analysis used in qualitative research, and to understand the relevance of qualitative research to occupational therapy, thereby enabling them to understand, analyse and critique published research articles.

Current changes within health care and rehabilitation are forcing corresponding changes in undergraduate education for the rehabilitation professions.

Recognition of the need for a client-centred approach to practice in order to tailor interventions appropriately and achieve (or at least strive for) accountability to our clients has demanded renewed attention to how we perform assessments (and what we deem appropriate to assess), how interventions may adhere to a client-centred model, and how outcomes can appropriately be evaluated. This reconsideration extends to curricular issues within rehabilitation education and the various tools provided to students to facilitate a client-centred service.

CLIENT-CENTRED PRACTICE

Client-centred practice has been defined as 'an approach to service which embraces a philosophy of respect for, and partnership with, people receiving services' (Law et al 1995, p. 253). The philosophy of client-centredness is central to occupational therapy in Canada (e.g. Canadian Association of Occupational Therapists 1991, 1997, Law 1998) and is a collaborative approach to intervention in which therapists 'demonstrate respect for clients, involve clients in decision making, advocate with and for clients in meeting clients' needs, and otherwise recognize clients' experience and knowledge' (Canadian Association of Occupational Therapists 1997, p. 49). Client-centred practice requires an emphasis on 'process': interaction, negotiation, education and exchange of information. In short, it is dependent upon communication (Hammell 1995).

Traditionally, knowledge deemed by the therapist to be objective or scientific (i.e. the therapist's knowledge) was accorded privilege over expertise derived from lived experience: the knowledge of the client. Client-centred practice attempts to utilize both forms of knowledge: the experiential knowledge of the client and the academic and practical knowledge of the therapist (Hammell 1998). This has led to an interest in qualitative forms of assessment and of narrative.

NARRATIVES IN REHABILITATION

A growing body of interdisciplinary literature suggests that narratives provide a powerful way of understanding human motives and actions (Helfrich et al 1994). They also provide a framework for understanding how the experience of disability (for example) is shaped within social and cultural frameworks, the significance of life events and the meaning of these for the client. This provides an insight into the client's goals and aspirations for the therapy programme.

Mishler (1986) observed that storytelling is usual in everyday conversation and that people will 'respond to questions with narratives if they are given some room to speak' (p. 69). Kielhofner and Mallinson (1995) provide some useful guidelines and suggestions for facilitating narratives within the context of acute-care or short-term treatment settings, demonstrating the utility of framing intervention around the client's perspective on their problems through the use of informal, semi-structured interviewing methods: giving clients the room to speak.

QUALITATIVE INTERVIEWING: ASSESSMENT AND OUTCOME 'MEASUREMENT'

Traditional forms of assessment within rehabilitation require the client to respond to standardized questions and predetermined categories deemed relevant by the therapist. Indeed, the literatures of our professions reveal a profusion of assessment tools and questionnaires. Although these forms of assessment are frequently deemed objective, it is important to recognize that '"objectivity" is not bestowed upon a measure merely because another person makes it' (Mor & Guadagnoli 1988, p. 1056): the categories deemed worthy of consideration reflect the values of those undertaking the assessment. They are not 'neutral' but value laden.

Therapists will treat what they assess; thus the assessment of abilities to perform certain self-care tasks, for example, will focus attention upon enhancement of those activities irrespective of their value to the individual (Hammell 1998), and clients have therefore been taught skills that are quickly discarded as irrelevant in the context of their everyday lives (e.g. Weingarden & Martin 1989, Yerxa & Locker 1990, Johnson 1993). Outcome measurement has reflected this therapist-centred view of the world: assessing the ability to perform skills that betray the values of the dominant culture (and which may reflect favourably upon the rehabilitation service) despite having little relevance to the individual.

Using qualitative methods in clinical interviewing

Occupational therapists and physical therapists are familiar with techniques of interviewing that are designed to glean 'pieces' of information deemed important by the therapist. A traditional interview might require the client to state, for example, the date of an injury, how it occurred, whether the client can perform transfers, climb stairs or dress independently.

In contrast, a more qualitative approach to interviewing might encourage a client to describe the impact of the injury upon their life, valued occupations and ability to enact social and family roles. Such an approach might incorporate open-ended questions which discourage typical 'yes' or 'no' responses, allowing the client's voice and perspectives to be heard. Thus, the aim would be to situate this particular illness, problem or injury within this particular life: an approach to interviewing that fits well with the client-centred orientation to rehabilitation advocated by contemporary theorists and therapists.

The Canadian Occupational Performance Measure (COPM; Law et al 1994) has been developed as a client-centred assessment tool. By prompting and facilitating a degree of narrativity, the COPM enables exploration of the client's life-world, values and goals, thereby providing the context for meaningful intervention and enhancing the possibility that the therapy programme will be directed towards the individual's life rather than their physical or emotional status.

It has been suggested that professional competence has two components: one is a sound grasp of the techniques or formal knowledge of the profession; the other is 'the ability to enter the patient's life-world so that the techniques are tailored to meet the patient's needs' (Crepeau 1991, p. 1024).

It is hoped that this brief exploration of client-centred practice and narrative will have

---

The life-world

Developed by philosophers Husserl and Schütz, the concept of the *life-world* constitutes the taken-for-granted, routine nature of everyday life: the 'realm of beliefs, assumptions, feelings, values, and cultural practices that constitute meaning in everyday life' (Kögler 1995, pp. 488–489).

explained the contemporary desire to situate therapy interventions within the context of individual lives, and that the need to seek qualitative information – the client's point of view – will be evident in this regard. However, it should be emphasized that the student assignment outlined in this chapter was grounded in a research, rather than a clinical context.

THE ETHNOGRAPHIC INTERVIEW

The student assignment discussed in this chapter focuses on an ethnographic interview: an interactive conversation with lines of questioning designed to probe specific areas of research interest. This semi-structured interview is informed by the questions and issues derived from the researcher's previous experience and knowledge, but is shaped situationally by reflecting upon the participant's evolving narrative. Primarily, the ethnographic interview is concerned with discovering the meaning of actions and events to the people whose lives we seek to understand (Spradley 1979).

McCracken (1988) suggests that the ethnographic or 'long' interview is one of the most powerful of qualitative methods, enabling insight into the life-world of the individual and the patterns and content of daily experience.

Although the students were asked to reflect upon how an ethnographic research interview differs from a clinical one, they also recognized and had the opportunity to experience the depth of information that may be elicited when qualitative interviewing techniques are used (and this is noted in the reflections on this interview assignment, below). The remainder of the chapter will explore and illustrate an undergraduate assignment designed to demonstrate the utility of this approach to interviewing.

THE ASSIGNMENT

After classes that addressed the qualitative research paradigm, research designs and

methods of data collection, the students were asked to conduct their own ethnographic interview with someone living in the community. Dr Dyck's instructions were as follows:

Choose a topic about which the person you are interviewing has experience and knowledge. You need to choose a topic that can provide you with information about how a person manages or makes sense of their day-to-day life. The person you interview will not normally be a close friend or relative with whom you have frequent contact.

The students were encouraged to select a topic that would enable them to explore another person's life from that person's perspective, rather than automatically to pursue a health- or disability-related issue. Initially, the choice of interviewee, the proposed topic for interview and three or four open-ended questions (to act as narrative stimulants) were discussed with the instructors to ensure suitability and relevance. Ethical procedures concerning informed consent and confidentiality were insisted upon, and the University's guidelines were followed in this regard.

The students were asked to keep notes on a number of issues, which would serve as the basis for subsequent class discussions as well as providing a framework for the written report. These questions were intended to encourage reflection on both the interview process and the influence of the students' social and personal positioning on the data. The students were asked to comment on the purpose of the interview and whether they obtained the information they had sought; how the interview participant was recruited; and a detailed description of the interview setting. They were requested to describe the interview process, including when it took place, how long it took, what preceded the 'formal' interview, the chosen method of recording, the rapport with the interviewee, and the issue of trust. Further, they were asked to consider any issues emerging from the interview which, if followed up in a research project, could enhance an understanding of any aspect of occupational therapy practice or theory. The emphasis of the assignment was on *process*: encouraging the students to focus primarily on the dynamics of the interviews, rather than solely upon the emerging data.

Despite heavy workloads and considerable pressure as their undergraduate education neared its conclusion, the students produced work that was both original and insightful, and which generated excitement and enthusiasm for this method of interviewing. The following sample of work by Toby Wendland provides a striking example of the ability of one student to glimpse the everyday life-world of another person and to portray this for a third person, the reader.

Although the students had not been asked to provide an analysis of their data, Toby had studied published reports of qualitative research that had been used as the basis for class discussions and undertook data analysis on his own initiative. His decisions regarding the selection, presentation and analysis of the data are both persuasive and compelling.

All names and places have been altered to preserve and protect the anonymity of Toby's informant. Acknowledging that the proposed use of 'Robert's' account in this chapter was not part of the initial consent contract agreed to between Robert and Toby, the context and purpose of this proposed chapter was fully explained to Robert and his permission sought. He willingly agreed to the inclusion of the piece, requested his own choice of pseudonym, and reviewed the chapter before it was submitted for publication. We are extremely grateful for his collaboration with this venture. What follows is Toby's unedited report of his interview.

ROBERT

Introduction

The purpose of the ethnographic interview was to determine what behaviours one gay male elementary school teacher has had to change while in his work environment because of his homosexuality. The interview had special relevance because he teaches in a fundamentalist Christian community. The behavioural changes he makes during such activities as parent–teacher interviews and teacher-to-teacher

interactions were focal questions in the interview. The interview also investigated what behaviours he must change in his day-to-day work activities with his grade seven students (12- and 13-year-olds) because of his sexual orientation. Through this process I also learned other ways in which his sexual orientation has affected his lifestyle outside the work environment.

Recruitment, trust and rapport

I recruited Robert (a pseudonym) for the interview because he was a long-time friend of my girlfriend, Marie. I had spoken with Robert several times in the preceding years, but never without Marie being present. Their relationship was the only reason I had ever interacted with Robert. Until this interview we had never spoken alone, aside from brief interactions. Without my relationship with Marie, I would not have accessed the opportunity to probe Robert's life in such detail. I am confident that Robert had trust in my professionalism with this issue because he had known for several years that I had no conscious prejudices against gay men. From previous discussions with Marie he also knew that I supported equal workplace and general societal rights for gay men. Likewise, he had known for several years through his understanding of Marie's values that she would never date a man who was prejudiced against gay men. For these reasons Robert understood my humanistic views toward homosexual people and appeared to trust me in the interview. This trust established good rapport between us and created a relaxed interview environment. It is noteworthy that as a teacher Robert is skilled in developing rapport; however, conversation seldom focuses on Robert and in this way the interview was a new experience.

Arranging the interview

I approached Robert about the interview over the phone approximately two weeks before it occurred. I explained to him that the purpose of the interview was to gain insight into the process involved in conducting an ethnographic interview. I told him my research questions at this time, primarily so he could make an informed decision about whether to participate in the interview, and secondly, so he would not be surprised when I asked him these questions during the interview. I assured him that all aspects of the interview would be kept confidential.

Positioning

There are many similarities between Robert and me that made rapport easy to establish, aside from the aforementioned issue of trust. We are both men in our twenties, with the same ethnic background, socio-economic status and level of education. Also, we were both born and raised in the same geographic region. Given these similarities, we have many similar values and can relate to and understand the circumstances affecting each other's lives. In comparison with my life, however, I learned from this interview that Robert's sexual orientation has affected his life in many complex and foreign ways. Since I am a heterosexual man, I view the issues with a different perspective and in this way my sexual orientation positions me as an outsider looking in.

Setting: the interviewer's participation in the interview

At Robert's request, I picked him up in my car the following morning at his home and together we went to a local family restaurant for breakfast. Both Robert and I had busy schedules and we agreed that the best use of our time would be to combine the interview with a meal. The family restaurant was chosen rather than a smaller (perhaps more fashionable), trendy restaurant because the latter typically has more crowded conditions and therefore less privacy. We sat in a booth in the back of the restaurant, since the tables for two were less private.

The restaurant was busy since we arrived for a late (10 am) breakfast. Once seated we initially spoke informally about work and school but the conversation then naturally moved to the interview topic. Robert looked a bit surprised when I asked him if I could tape the interview, but he consented given that the tape would be erased after the paper was written. My participation in the interview was active in that whenever possible I spontaneously added questions to enrich and promote Robert's opportunity to speak freely, but he did 90% of the talking while I actively listened. Robert controlled the majority of the interaction by speaking on what he thought was important. Robert provided many valuable comments that gave greater insight into his work life as a gay man than could have been possible if I had dominated the interview. For example, after Robert had finished a general description of a topical area, he would illustrate other areas that would help clarify his position without requiring prompting. The taped portion of the interview took approximately 45 minutes, but the entire time together from pick-up to drop off was an hour and fifteen minutes.

Findings of the interview

The next section of the paper reports the findings of the interview based upon analysis of the data

recordings. Data was recorded and analysed from an audio recording of the interview and from field notes made immediately after dropping Robert off at his home. I was able to identify two categories in the data: (1) effects upon behaviour within the work environment (physical separation from work to assure anonymity with partner, teacher-to-teacher interactions and interactions with parents/student; (2) effects upon behaviour within non-work environments (avoidance and relationships, social events).

1. Effects upon behaviour within the work environment

Physical separation from work to assure anonymity with partner. Robert's residence and the restaurant are over 110 kilometres from the community and school in which he teaches: it is very important to Robert that no one from his school environment sees him with his partner. In the previous years I had learned that Robert chose to live far away from his job because he wanted to lessen the chance of someone from his school environment (staff, parents, or students) knowing anything about his personal life. Robert chooses to keep his homosexual identity hidden in his professional life for important reasons. One reason is that he wishes to move into school administration. Robert must keep his homosexuality a secret because he believes the political and social forces within the school system will not allow a gay man to attain such a high position of authority. After asking Robert how his homosexuality affects his professional goals he explained:

> I want to go into administration, probably, ... you know vice principal or principal. I'd like to be a part in that, but I know or I assume that my chances of getting it if it was known that I was gay would make it a lot more difficult. For whatever reason, even though they might think I'd be a good administrator, it would probably be difficult to justify it to the parents.

Teacher-to-teacher interactions. Even when people from work reach out with a helping hand to offer support in difficult times Robert must be careful. During his first year of teaching, Robert had not told anyone of his homosexuality and as a result he described that year as 'very miserable'. He must have appeared quite 'down' while at work because another teacher offered to help him. Robert could not accept the teacher's help because he could not let his identity be known:

> I was very, very unhappy during that time and near the end of the year one of the [teachers]

said, 'I hope you're able to sort through whatever you're going through right now'. He was a really nice guy, and went to church and everything, and he asked if we'd like to go out for lunch or something. But I obviously could never have told him. He was a fundamentalist guy and there's no way I could have told him. Who knows what he might have said? It could've been good or bad. I wasn't willing to take that chance.

It has become a habit that Robert avoids conversations that focus on him because such conversation can easily lead to personal topics that might give clues about his homosexuality. Robert noted that he has become adept in skilfully circumnavigating conversations that may lead to revealing facts about his personal life:

I'm very careful about how I discuss it. I don't bring conversations up like that where there'll be people asking me questions ... The pressure is always there. The thing is that you're always automatically justifying or getting around conversations so it doesn't lead to that ... I was out the other night with this new woman on staff; she's a teacher and, you know, there's the question, 'So, are you seeing anybody?' And I said, 'Yes', and then she says, 'Well how did you meet her?', and I said, 'Well, we were playing tennis', and you don't ever say 'he' or 'she'. I just didn't want to discuss it. What I saw happening was that I was giving such short answers that she figured out something and stopped asking questions. Anyway the conversation shifted to her husband, and I quickly moved on to something else.

Robert described the unseen differences that put him under unique social pressures within the work environment:

For example, at work you have to give an emergency phone contact name and number. At my last school I had Marie down, and I thought, 'This is crazy! I can't keep doing this'. To a degree it's paranoia; I mean just because I have another guy on there doesn't mean I'm gay. But my problem is that – well – that [the male 'emergency contact'] is just one more thing so that if someone suspects something's going on it's just going to lead to that [that workers will discover he is gay]. This time I did put [partner's name] down and underneath, under 'relationship' I just put 'friend' ... When I moved in with [partner] I got a separate phone line so when people phoned they'd get my machine and they'd get my voice on it ... As far as they would know

there would be no one else living there ... I'm very careful about who I tell [about his homosexuality] ... Stuff like that – that would not normally be an issue to anybody – you have to be aware of all the time.

Interactions with parents/students. A second issue within the work environment related to the special care Robert has to take in order to conceal his homosexuality from parents and students:

Parents watch your every move. Parents are a major stress to me in my job. Kids; I deal with any hard-core problem if it's with them. Grade sevens (aged about 12) always want to know everything about you, and they always ask, 'Are you married? and I say, 'No'. With sexual education that I'll be teaching this year, I'll have to be very careful when I answer touchy questions not to be one sided or show anything that could give them a hint that I'm gay. If a kid goes home and says, 'Mr Robert says it's OK to be a homosexual', and this kid's dad's a redneck ['redneck' refers to someone who demonstrates widely discriminative behaviours and is generally unaccepting of people's differences], then I could be in for some big trouble. It's always having to be careful about what might lead to what.

2. Effects upon behaviour within non-work environments

Avoidance and relationships. To many friends, Robert appears to have a shy personality and a possible reason for this is that he seldom talks about himself. In fact, it is more accurate to describe Robert as quiet when he is around people he does not know well. Much of Robert's shy personality has developed over the years since he began to realize he was gay. The results of hiding his sexuality during his early adolescence, teen years and early adulthood has shaped his behaviours to create a quiet, or apparently shy personality.

He related some of his memories of behaviours he chose to modify in order to hide his homosexuality. Robert commented on high school and how it set a pattern of avoidance:

By 13 or 14 you're expected to have a girlfriend. It's just what happens. I even had girlfriends but after two or three times of things never going very far [physically] (because I was never that interested) you just don't bother with it any more [dating women]. People are watching and waiting for it. Girls would come on to you and what are you supposed to do? It was a difficult time. I never had any other relationships from then on until I got to the city. People start to say, 'Well, what's up with him?' When that starts you're like, 'I have to get away from this'. And that's when I started to go from place to place. I'd have a group of friends and it would be apparent after too long that I didn't have a girlfriend or whatever. Then I'd move on to something else. I was at university for two years and then I went back to my home community; and then I had a new group of friends. Then I went back to the city and met a whole new group of friends.

Thus Robert chose to stop having personal relationships and avoided establishing long-term friendships. Avoidance also affected his participation in normal peer activities when he was in his formative years:

Another example, especially when I was younger was that I could never get drunk because, you know, what would happen if I got in a situation where I started saying things about who I really was? Take university for example. You know, the guys are all out watching strippers or in a bar or whatever. They're checking out women and stuff like that and saying, 'Hey, look at her!' or whatever, and of course I just went along with it.

Robert explained how he kept his identity hidden from two good friends. While living in the city he would not let the two friends come in contact with each other. Each was from a different window in his life: one he knew from high school and the other from university. His fear was that if either of them had the opportunity to combine their knowledge they would deduce that Robert was gay. He recounts: 'I kept aspects of my life separate'.

Social events. At present, social events like weddings continually pose difficult situations for Robert. Robert stated that, 'People always say stuff [at weddings] like, "Oh, you still don't have a girlfriend!" and it's hard to respond to if you want to keep quiet'. Having fellow workers come over to one's house would be a social event Robert would really enjoy but he cannot let this happen:

It would be really nice to have people over from work. Or for example, after work everybody else is calling their boyfriend, husbands or wives. And I can never do that. I have to sneak off and use a pay phone to call [my partner]. It would be nice for us all [the teachers] to go out for a beer and for me to be able to invite him. But it's not going to happen.

Anger

When asked if hiding his identity made him angry, Robert replied:

Yeah, it bugs me. I have a lot of anger actually. I feel ripped off in a lot of ways. Stuff that straight people can take for granted. Like calling someone to meet you, or going out with friends from work, with other couples or whatever. I can't have it. I can't do that. I mean I could, but it would mean dealing with a lot of other stuff. It totally changes your life in aspects that straight people would never think of and actually take for granted.

When I added that Robert's feelings were much like those cited by people with disabilities, Robert said:

Not that in any way would I want to have a physical disability or whatever, but at least if you have that then generally it's obvious and people are aware of it that in some way it [the disability] is going to change your life. People would acknowledge it and I can't have that at all. And I would have really liked to have had kids. That really bugs me. I wouldn't do it because of the social reaction the kids might have to deal with.

In this way it appears that Robert feels he has an invisible disability in that he cannot do the things he wants because society will not permit it without a drastic cost.

Enhancing the quality of data

The interview may have provided higher quality data if we had gone out for a coffee. Conducting the interview over a meal may have made Robert feel somewhat uncomfortable because I had finished my breakfast long before he finished his, and he therefore may have felt a little pressure to eat more and talk less. Although I tried to encourage him to speak freely, my plate was removed from the table and Robert was left with half a plate of food to eat while I sipped the remains of a cup of coffee. As Robert had felt that going out for breakfast was the ideal situation, however, I believe that confronting his idea would have only emphasized the inevitable power inequalities between the interviewer and subject. Another possible alternative could have been for me to eat my food more slowly so that we both would have finished our meals together.

Recording the conversation may have also affected the data. It is possible that Robert may not have said all he would have if I had not recorded the conversation. Asking Robert about the tape recorder during my initial phone conversation could have given him greater power to choose not to be recorded. If he had known about the plan to record him earlier (and agreed to it), he could have chosen to withhold more information. Conversely, more time could have enabled him to be more emotionally prepared.

Reflecting upon the qualitative process

The process of conducting this ethnographic interview, analysing the data and writing the paper has reinforced the research concepts used in the qualitative research process. Although I believed I understood Robert thoroughly upon the finish of the interview, it was only after multiple analyses of the recordings and field notes that I was able to uncover a greater richness of information. At the outset of the interview my plan had been to have my prime research questions answered, along with the expectation that the free nature of the interview would allow Robert to provide an inside (or emic) perspective upon the chosen topic. The discovery of the categories and subcategories within the data required several separate analyses.

Upon the completion of the interview I believed that I had a clear picture of what Robert had said. A second analysis occurred after the cassette tape was transcribed onto paper and then scrutinized in the search for themes and categories of data. At this point, while on the computer, the data seemed fractured and it was difficult to assimilate passages in order to identify predominant themes. The third analysis occurred as the paper was physically laid out upon the floor to match (or rebut) my perceived concepts with actual quotes from the interview. Only after trying to utilize quotes to support my interpretations of the meanings of Robert's responses, however, did I realize the complexity of human interaction and the tremendous effort required to derive meaning from words alone. Most interesting was how the categories seemed to unfold from the data in an inductive manner, whereas until then they had been only theoretical concepts. Upon a peer review by my colleagues a fourth analysis uncovered further data – construct linkages. The additional consideration of reflexivity added to my overall view of the epistemological impact upon qualitative research methodology. My perception at the outset that Robert willingly accepted the personal nature of the interview topics was supported during the final analysis when he read through the paper. Robert reported that the data–construct linkages accurately reflected his own feelings about that aspect of his life. This final phase of the analysis helped to assure the quality of the data.

Further OT research

How a man's sexual orientation can affect his activities of daily living, especially in relation to work behaviour, is an area that occupational therapists need to consider. This interview has provided examples that portray how the effects of social alienation due to sexual orientation can hinder a man's ability to maximize his productivity and live a fulfilling life. Understanding why one homosexual man has chosen to hide an important aspect of his self-identity in order to assure success in the professional teaching arena can help raise the OT's awareness of the importance of being sensitive to sexual issues. In turn, OTs must consider the far-reaching effects of how clients may change their behaviour to hide their sexual orientation. The wide ramifications homosexuality may have upon the client can hinder the effectiveness of occupational therapy when clients feel they have to camouflage their sexual orientation. As exemplified in this interview, the behaviours and cognitive strategies clients may be obliged to employ in order to hide their true identity can cause significant emotional and cognitive stress. These stresses surely have a negative effect on life satisfaction.

The lifestyle changes one gay man has been forced to develop as a result of his sexuality illustrate the complexity of his interactions with his social, cultural, and physical environments. In terms of OT, for example, consider the extra stress that clients may experience when a therapist is trying to build therapeutic rapport, or trying to assess social support networks, when homosexual clients are trying to hide their sexual orientation. Such an issue could certainly be present in any physical or mental health field of occupational therapy practice. More ethnographic research into this area is needed to better affirm and clarify the effects of sexual orientation upon behaviour so that occupational therapy can better acknowledge and address the problems facing homosexual clients.

Acknowledgements

I would like to thank Robert for his participation in this ethnographic research paper.

REFLECTIONS

Almost 2 years after this student assignment, I asked Toby to reflect upon it again in light of his subsequent experience of working as an occupational therapist in the United States. Here are his reflections.

As a practising occupational therapist, the information I learned from conducting an ethnographic interview has made me more sensitive to the client's point of view. In turn, hearing clients' and families' stories with an open mind continues to help me derive more succinct and client-centred goals. My challenge, however, is to successfully blend the non-therapeutic factors in the work environment (primarily economic and bureaucratic) with the therapeutic or clinical factors to create a good therapeutic milieu.

I gained insights into many clients' illness experiences from the ethnographic approach that would have been impossible if I had come to the interview with a standardized, medical model style of interview. Integrating this style of interview has enhanced my ability and opportunity to gain client rapport and establish trust. The ethnographic approach has improved my ability to collect the right data and integrate it into a client-centred plan of intervention. In this way I look deeper into my own interaction with clients and question more deeply my own hypotheses and clinical reasoning.

The challenge of integrating the ethnographic interview is to establish a balance between the requirements of the clinical work environment and striving to achieve the idealism learned during my OT education. At university I internalized a clinical reasoning model where my main goal was to establish client-centred treatment. At work, however, limited time and resources restrict my ability effectively to collect subjective information from every client with a qualitative approach.

Even with all the imperfections occasioned by working within an organization, the experience of conducting the ethnographic interview has given me the skills to analyse my own prejudices and preconceived notions when I practise therapy.

REFERENCES

Canadian Association of Occupational Therapists 1991 Occupational therapy guidelines for client centred practice. CAOT Publications, Toronto

Canadian Association of Occupational Therapists 1997 Enabling occupation. An occupational therapy perspective. Canadian Association of Occupational Therapists, Ottawa

Crepeau EB 1991 Achieving intersubjective understanding: examples from an occupational therapy treatment session. American Journal of Occupational Therapy 45(11):1016–1025

Hammell KW 1995 Spinal cord injury rehabilitation. Chapman & Hall, London

Hammell KW 1998 Client-centred occupational therapy: collaborative planning, accountable intervention. In: Law M (ed) Client-centered occupational therapy. Slack, New Jersey, pp 123–143

Helfrich C, Kielhofner G, Mattingly C 1994 Volition as narrative: understanding motivation in chronic illness. American Journal of Occupational Therapy 48(4):311–317

Johnson R 1993 'Attitudes don't just hang in the air …' Disabled people's perceptions of physical therapists. Physiotherapy 79(9):619–626

Kielhofner G, Mallinson T 1995 Gathering narrative data through interviews: empirical observations and suggested guidelines. Scandinavian Journal of Occupational Therapy 2:63–68

Kögler H-H 1995 The life world. In: Honderich T (ed) The Oxford companion to philosophy. Oxford University Press, Oxford, pp 488–489

Law M 1998 Client-centered occupational therapy. Slack, New Jersey

Law M, Baptiste S, Carswell A, McColl MA, Polatajko H, Pollock N 1994 Canadian Occupational Performance Measure: 2nd edn. CAOT Publications, Toronto

Law M, Baptiste S, Mills J 1995 Client-centred practice: what does it mean and does it make a difference? Canadian Journal of Occupational Therapy 62:250–257

McCracken G 1988 The long interview. Sage, Newbury Park

Mishler EG 1986 Research interviewing. Context and narrative. Harvard University Press, Cambridge, MA

Mor V, Guadagnoli E 1988 Quality of life measurement: a psychometric Tower of Babel. Journal of Clinical Epidemiology 41(11):1055–1058

Spradley JP 1979 The ethnographic interview. Harcourt Brace Jovanovich, Orlando

Weingarden SI, Martin C 1989 Independent dressing after spinal cord injury: a functional time evaluation. Archives of Physical Medicine and Rehabilitation 70:518–519

Yerxa EJ, Locker SB 1990 Quality of time use by adults with spinal cord injuries. American Journal of Occupational Therapy 44(4):318–326

FURTHER READING

Holstein JA, Gubrium JF 1995 The active interview. Sage, Thousand Oaks

Spencer J, Krefting L, Mattingly C 1993 Incorporation of ethnographic methods in occupational therapy assessment. American Journal of Occupational Therapy 47(4):303–309

Evaluating qualitative research

Chris Carpenter   *Karen Hammell*

OVERVIEW

In this chapter we will discuss general evaluative criteria that have been specifically developed to enhance the rigour and plausibility of qualitative research. The chapter is intended to provide researchers and consumers of research with the background needed to ascertain the merits of a research study. With this in mind we have provided a framework of evaluative guidelines which will, we hope, assist readers critically to read and assess our professional literatures.

GENERAL CRITERIA FOR EVALUATION OF RESEARCH

Criteria for assessing the quality and merit of research have long been an integral component of quantitative research design. The struggle to establish the trustworthiness or merit of qualitative research is ongoing, and can best be understood by briefly revisiting the relationship between the qualitative and quantitative paradigms (this was explored by Lyn Jongbloed in Chapter 2).

> *Inductive reasoning*: using observation to formulate an idea or theory.
>
> *Deductive reasoning*: taking a known idea or theory and applying it to a situation.
>
> (Clifford 1997, p.10)

Quantitative research: assumptions and evaluation

Quantitative research is characterized by a formal, systematic process in which numerical data are used to quantify or measure relationships between phenomena and produce statistical findings. Also referred to as 'positivism' or 'empiricism', it describes, tests and examines cause-and-effect relationships, using a deductive process of knowledge attainment (Clifford 1997).

Judgements about good research in this tradition are closely referenced to methodology; prescribed strategies are thus employed to enhance rigour and are assessed through reference to criteria supporting reliability, internal and external validity, and generalizability of both the data and data collection methods, and of the measurement tools. By examining hypothesized relationships and proposing interpretations, the quantitative approach tests theory deductively from existing knowledge.

Mays and Pope (1995) observed that 'As in quantitative research, the basic strategy to ensure rigour in qualitative research is systematic and self conscious research design, data collection, interpretation, and communication' (p. 110). However, the different assumptions that underlie quantitative and qualitative approaches demand different strategies to ensure rigour and quality in the research process and subsequent inferences.

Qualitative research: assumptions and evaluation

Qualitative approaches have in common the desire to study the world from the perspective of the study participants, not the researcher (Domholdt 1993). As a result, qualitative researchers do not begin their inquiry with a researcher-developed hypothesis, but rather with certain ideas, perspectives or hunches that may be important in shaping and understanding the research. In this way qualitative approaches develop theory inductively.

Recognition of the role of qualitative research in contributing to knowledge within the medical and rehabilitation disciplines has traditionally been inhibited by a lack of published papers. For those interested in pursuing or publishing qualitative research, concerns are raised that funding bodies or reviewers of articles submitted for publication have an inadequate grounding in qualitative inquiry and a bias towards positivism, and are therefore unable to provide informed assessments of the merits of qualitative research (Gliner 1994). As Krefting (1991) pointed out, 'too frequently, qualitative research is evaluated against criteria appropriate to quantitative research and is found to be lacking' (p. 214). This is not due to an inherent inadequacy, but rather to the inappropriate imposition of criteria developed for a different form of inquiry. (Of course, to assess quantitative research by qualitative criteria would produce similar misunderstandings.) It has become clear that the nature and purpose of the two research traditions are different, but not necessarily exclusive (for example, see Chapter 2). The nature and purpose of their respective evaluative criteria, however, remain distinct.

Rigour and ethics

Given the pluralistic nature of qualitative inquiry, not all qualitative research can be evaluated using the same criteria or strategies. As Sandelowski (1986) noted, the term 'qualitative research' is imprecise and refers to many dissimilar research methods (see Chapter 1). Agar (1986) suggested that a different language is needed to fit the qualitative view, and advocated that reliability and validity be replaced by alternative concepts.

Atkinson (1990) suggested the general categories of authenticity and plausibility as a means of evaluating qualitative research. These incorporate much of the four evaluative criteria (credibility, transferability, dependability and confirmability) proposed some years earlier by Lincoln and Guba (1985). Dictionary definitions of *authenticity* suggest qualities such as genuine, authoritative; something that is, in fact, as represented, reliable, trustworthy and of established credibility. The concept of authenticity turns the evaluative spotlight on to the researcher as the key research instrument (Bogdan & Biklen 1998) and demands a full account of their positionality, both biographical and philosophical. It is these positionalities that will affect the degree of engagement with the subject matter and participants, and will also, by default, affect data collection, analysis and theoretical sensitivity, as these dimensions stand in reciprocal relationships with each other (Strauss & Corbin 1990). *Plausibility* is concerned with determining whether 'the findings of the study, whether in the form of description, explanation, or theory, "fit" the data from which they are derived' (Sandelowski 1986, p. 32). This general criterion focuses on the evaluation of the data collection methods and whether enough information is available to allow the reader to judge the adequacy of the research process. Plausibility also seeks to evaluate the linkages between the data and the reported findings. As Atkinson (1990) suggests, 'if they [the findings] are to be recognized as authoritative then they must persuade the reader of their plausibility' (p. 175). Acker, Barry and Esseveld (1991) propose in addition that researchers ensure the participants' voices are heard, accounting for the researchers' viewpoints as well as those of the participants, and revealing the contextual issues inherent in the daily lives of those being studied.

The development of criteria that will support the merit of qualitative research can be likened to a work in progress. Like all research, qualitative research is influenced by political and ethical issues at the societal, institutional and professional levels. Punch (1994) identifies three developments that have exerted a significant influence on our awareness of the ethical dimensions of research. First, feminist scholarship that emphasizes identification, trust, empathy and non-exploitative relationships. Second, the movement towards interventionist work or 'action' research, which emphasizes the central role of study participants as partners in the research process and which demands attention to the purpose or outcome of the research; and third, the heightened concern on the part of governments and institutions with informed consent and confidentiality: an issue that affects the research review process, funding and involvement of participants.

Guba (1981) had originally proposed the criteria of trustworthiness and authenticity, but was clear that these 'should not be reconstituted into an orthodoxy' (p. 90). There is an inherent tension 'between the creativity of the qualitative research process – which implies contingent methods to capture the richness of context-dependent sites and situations – and evaluation – which implies standardized procedures and modes of reporting' (Baxter & Eyles 1997, p. 505). Accordingly, we advocate seeking reference to general strategies, to enhance rigour and ensure meaningful inferences from research, rather than to a set of rigid rules, suggesting that these criteria serve as 'anchor points' (Baxter & Eyles 1997, p. 505) for the evaluation of qualitative research.

STRATEGIES TO EVALUATE THE RIGOUR OF QUALITATIVE INQUIRY

Growing interest in qualitative methodologies as legitimate approaches to research questions in the social sciences and health-care disciplines has created a need for conceptual models to assess the merits of such research (Krefting 1991). A number of strategies have been identified that can be used by qualitative researchers in their efforts to enhance the rigour of their studies. Some need to be incorporated in the study design phase, others during data collection, analysis, or after the study has been completed and the research is written up. An understanding of these strategies will assist the reader to critically read published research studies that have used a qualitative research design.

It is important to remember that these strategies need to be appropriately selected for specific studies: not all are appropriate to every qualitative study. We propose a review of potential strategies to enhance the rigour of qualitative inquiry using the following criteria (adapted from Baxter & Eyles 1997):

- Provision of information on the appropriateness of the methodology
- Use of multiple methods and the reasons for each choice (triangulation)
- Information on participant selection
- Details of how interviews were conducted
- The researcher's role is critically examined (reflexivity/positionality)
- Presentation of verbatim quotations
- Description of how data were converted into theoretical constructs
- Length of time spent in fieldwork is stated
- Relating current findings to existing theories
- Revisits to respondents to clarify meanings and verify interpretations
- Attention to power relations involved in data collection process
- Ethical implications of representation and publication.

Provision of information on the appropriateness of the methodology

In Chapter 1 we indicated that qualitative and quantitative research methods are useful for different sorts of questions, proposing that the choice of a research methodology should be informed by the nature of the problem it seeks to address. Accordingly, any research study should be evaluated on the degree to which the choice of methodology 'fits' the issue under study. This includes consideration of the original purpose of the research and a rationale for the selected methodology.

Use of multiple methods and the reasons for each choice

Plausibility may be assessed by determining whether the researcher obtained sufficient data and whether any degree of triangulation was used. *Triangulation* is based on the premise that the convergence of a number of perspectives will confirm the data obtained and ensure that all aspects of the phenomenon have been investigated. This strategy can take a range of forms: the use of multiple sources, multiple methods or multiple investigators (Krefting 1991).

Source triangulation may be achieved by using multiple informants, to corroborate, elaborate or illuminate the phenomenon under study (Marshall & Rossman 1989) and by using more than one report from a data set to corroborate a construct (Baxter & Eyles 1997).

Another common method involves comparing data generated by different collection methods. Melinda Suto (Chapter 4) describes how she obtained data from a number of sources over a prolonged period of time. These sources, which included participant observation, ethnographic interviews and facility documents, enabled a richer and deeper understanding of how people with chronic schizophrenia use time and the environment to enact their daily occupations.

However, simply using more than one method does not necessarily guarantee more rigorous results. Baxter and Eyles (1997) observe that few researchers comment on the reasons for the use of several methods, explain whether they feel these address the same or different questions, or explore the implications of any discrepancies in data emanating from multiple sources. Further, Hasselkus (1991) notes that triangulation of methods may not be appropriate or applicable in every instance; for example, a researcher may place greater emphasis upon interviews than upon prolonged observation, if observation is viewed as being too intrusive and unnecessary to the central purpose of the research.

Triangulation can also be achieved by expanding the range of data that might contribute to an understanding of the phenomenon. Krefting (1991) suggests that in a hospital setting, for example, this might involve observing different shifts on different wards, or focus on patients, family and professionals, either alone or in small groups. (For example, the strategy of enhancing understanding by interviewing both members of a couple is demonstrated by Sue Stanton in Chapter 5.)

The involvement of more than one investigator can also be viewed as a form of triangulation. In Chapter 7 Sue Forwell describes how two primary researchers and a research assistant collaborated to formulate interview questions and analyse data. The involvement of a number of researchers is sometimes seen as an advantage in that the research process is enriched by a diversity of perspectives.

Peer review

Researchers are encouraged to solicit the help of colleagues who have experience with qualitative methods in reviewing field notes and transcripts to see whether they identify the same categories and themes within the data as the researcher: a further instance of triangulation. Chris Carpenter (Chapter 3) asked a colleague to identify units of meaning from the interview transcripts and to assign them to categories that were beginning to emerge, using the definitions she had established. The reviewer brought a new perspective to the data, and as a result Carpenter was required clearly to articulate her reasoning, and more clearly define the categories she had developed. As Lincoln and Guba (1985) suggest, peer review is one way of keeping the researcher honest, and the searching questions that result may contribute to a deeper reflexive analysis. However, it is important to emphasize that peer examination is designed to help clarify the researcher's perspectives: the colleague does not represent a standard against which the findings are compared (Hasselkus 1991); nor is this an attempt to obtain a second opinion, as there are real dangers 'that one person may defer to the other on the basis of unequal power/relations' (Baxter & Eyles 1997, p. 514). Publication of the study findings can be seen as a retrospective form of peer review. It is therefore essential that articles submitted for publication include rich excerpts from primary field notes and interview transcripts, and an in-depth explanation of the decisions made during the research process. In other words, it must be possible for the reader to follow the decision trail of the researcher in terms of their development of concepts, presentation of arguments, and construct–data linkages.

Information on participant selection

The plausibility of a study may be partially assessed through reference to the study participants: whether the method of sampling was relevant and appropriate; whether the sample relates to the group of which they are members; and whether a bias occurred due to either sampling or access. (This refers to instances where the method of sampling has led the researcher to a group of people who share similar viewpoints, but which would not necessarily reflect the larger group of which they are members.) This requires information concerning how participants were recruited and how many people were interviewed (and the reasons for this number). Sampling may be random or purposeful, depending upon the nature and purpose of the study. Certain methods of selection, such as snowball sampling or convenience sampling, may lead the researcher to easy contacts who do not represent or reflect the larger group from which they are drawn, yet these methods may be perfectly well suited to accessing certain study populations (for example, see Chapter 6). The sample may be selected serially or continuously focused and selected in response to the concurrent analysis of emerging data, in an effort to search for negative cases and enhance the depth of data (Baxter & Eyles 1997).

Research reports could usefully consider the limitations imposed by the selected sampling strategy, providing a database that enables the reader to determine whether the findings from one situation might be applicable ('transferable') to another situation that is sufficiently similar (although a multisite study is most likely to enable transferability of study findings; Baxter & Eyles 1997). Further, a description of participant characteristics is critical in offering 'an indication of who is allowed to speak and, of equal importance, who is not' (Baxter & Eyles 1997, p. 508). This issue of 'voice' will be addressed again.

Details of how interviews were conducted

Some detail should be provided concerning the data collection process. Research credibility can be enhanced within the interviewing process, for example, by such strategies as reframing or expanding questions (Krefting 1991). Some researchers elect to narrow their inquiry progressively, responding to the narratives of the participants to 'funnel' the subject matter of the interviews. Other researchers are guided by a basic checklist of issues and enable every participant to cover the same topics, allowing them the freedom to elaborate or describe their experience without being constrained by an increasingly narrow framework of inquiry (Baxter and Eyles 1997). This enables any discrepant views, differing opinions or 'negative cases' (Gliner 1994) to be identified and addressed. Such strategies should be delineated for the reviewer.

Central to data collection is the means of capturing information: what is the method of record keeping? This should be noted. Usually, interviews will be audiotaped and transcribed. This eliminates the need to take notes during the interviews and enables the researcher to capture and preserve the conversations in their entirety for subsequent in-depth analysis or peer review.

Field notes are recorded immediately after concluding each interview, as a means to document perceptions and impressions, the

---

> **Box 10.1** Suggested checklist for recording field notes (Adapted from Morse JM, Field PA Qualitative research methods for health professionals, p. 115, copyright © 1995 by Sage Publications. Reprinted by permission of Sage Publications, Inc.)
>
> ◆ Interview date, start time, ending time
> ◆ Pre-interview goals
> ◆ Location of the interview
> ◆ Description of the environment (e.g. physical space, equipment)
> ◆ People present (any activities? interactions?)
> ◆ Content of interview (key words, topics, focus, what stood out?)
> ◆ Non-verbal behaviour (voice, posture, eyes, gestures?)
> ◆ Researcher's impressions (discomfort with any topics? emotional responses?)
> ◆ Technological problems? (did the tape recorder work!)
> ◆ Impact of researcher positioning (positive or negative?)
> ◆ Analysis (questions, hunches, familiar themes, data trends, emerging patterns?)

dynamics of the interaction and any problems encountered. Headings may facilitate the process of recording field notes. Box 10.1 illustrates a suggested checklist for recording field notes.

Further, many researchers maintain a diary to record feelings and ideas about the research, including any problems, discrepancies or gaps in the information being generated. This provides an opportunity to monitor progress, and to compare ideas and data with theoretical concepts that might help to explain them.

It is important to state clearly who undertook the interviews. In some instances research assistants undertake all the face-to-face contact with study participants, perhaps because of issues of confidentiality (for example, see Sue Forwell's discussion in Chapter 7) or because of language incompatibility. These reasons should be stated, as they are part of a clear research strategy (and may thus be differentiated from more problematic instances, where researchers use assistants to save themselves time and effort).

All these dimensions of the data collection and research processes must be documented clearly to enhance the credibility of the research and the plausibility of the findings.

The researcher's role is critically examined (reflexivity/positionality)

The concept of *positionality* is related to the imperative to make transparent the research relationship, as this affects both process and purpose (this is explored by Chris Carpenter in Chapter 3, and by Karen Hammell in Chapter 6). It has been proposed that, in understanding qualitative research, the researcher is the key research instrument (e.g. Bogdan & Biklen 1998). To accept this proposition is to necessitate a critical evaluation of the position of the researcher with respect to the particular study.

The issue of positioning should be carefully examined by the researcher – and made evident for the reader – in relation to such issues as to what extent the research process, write-up and dissemination of the findings deals with the relationships between the researcher and the participants, and between the researcher and the academic community in terms of power dynamics and veracity. These are issues that pertain to 'where one speaks from' (recognizing that we all speak 'from' our perspective as the member of a particular gender, sexual identity, class, ethnicity and so forth): what Alcoff (1991) terms our 'location'. According to Alcoff, location affects the meaning and context of what one says: one cannot assume an ability to transcend one's 'social' location or social identity.

Qualitative researchers consider it unrealistic to postulate the elimination of the researcher as a person from the research process. Oakley (1981) calls this 'the mythology of "hygienic" research with its accompanying mystification of the researcher and the researched as objective instruments of data collection' (p. 58). Her central premise is that scientific detachment 'be replaced by the recognition that personal involvement is more than dangerous bias – it is the condition under which people come to know each other and to admit others into their lives' (p. 58): involvement is not undesirable, it is essential to an ethical relationship.

The concept of *reflexivity* is a response to a concern with 'bias', which is viewed by qualitative researchers as being a misplaced term. Rather than biases, various positionalities are seen as resources that are used by researchers to guide data gathering and to understand their own interpretations and behaviour in research (Olesen 1994). Reflexivity entails articulation of the deep-seated (but often poorly recognized) views and judgements that affect the research topic, including a full assessment of the influence of the researcher's background, perceptions and interests on the research process. Thus, in describing her own role as researcher, Chris Carpenter (Chapter 3) explained how it was both impossible and undesirable to claim neutrality, given her extensive clinical practice in spinal cord injury rehabilitation and her friendships with individuals who had sustained such injuries; rather, this formed the background from which she designed and implemented the study. Self-reflexivity, employed with integrity throughout the research process, may also reveal, for example, how a theory held by the researcher at the beginning of the research process has been challenged or changed as a result of the data. However, it has been observed that researchers only rarely mention their motivations, biases and interests in relation to the questions asked and decisions made during the research process (Baxter & Eyles 1997), yet these dimensions of the researcher role need to be explicitly stated for the reader in order to contribute to the overall trustworthiness of the research.

Presentation of verbatim quotations

Quotations are important 'for revealing how meanings are expressed in the respondents' own words rather than the words of the researcher' (Baxter & Eyles 1997, p. 508). However, while some researchers provide many quotes with little accompanying commentary, others provide few quotes with considerable commentary; thus the reader must judge whether the provided quotations support the researcher's interpretations and whether the quotations are, indeed, representative of common themes. Further, there must always be recognition that quotations are, of necessity, anecdotal. In addition, the selection of some words and not others, the voices of some participants and not others represents the power of researchers vis-à-vis the research process and the choices made based on their understandings and agendas. Again, these choices should be made clear.

Description of how data were converted into theoretical constructs

The researcher needs to provide some comment on the procedures used for data analysis. Baxter and Eyles (1997) claim that 'it is necessary to elaborate how data get transformed into concepts/theory(ies) to show readers whose meanings are represented and why' (p. 509).

Plausibility may be partially assessed through a consideration of the proportion of data that has been taken into account in the process of analysis and interpretation. The reader must be able to judge whether some information has been ignored or overlooked if it failed to fit a chosen theoretical or interpretive framework. An audit trail should enable the reader to determine whether enough information has been provided to judge the adequacy of the research process and, further, to assess whether interpretations flow from the data rather than being imposed on them (Robson 1993). Thus, readers should be able to follow the progression of the research and determine whether the interpretations are justified, or indeed plausible.

In instances where research assistants have been used to generate interview data, it should be indicated that the researcher is interpreting those data in the absence of interaction – the 'relationship' dimension usually considered so central to qualitative research – and the implications of this remoteness from the research participants must be subject to critical analysis.

Baxter and Eyles (1997) note that the dependability of interpretations in qualitative research may be threatened by poorly defined analytical constructs. They suggest some strategies which may enhance dependability, including mechanical recording of data (to enable accurate comparisons with the data), participant researchers and peer examination.

Length of time spent in fieldwork is stated

Melinda Suto's study (Chapter 4) illustrates the benefits of 'prolonged engagement', which allowed the participants (in this study the residents of the board and care home) to become accustomed to the presence of the researcher and which afforded the opportunity to confirm the data over time. Data collection over a period of time has the advantage of decreasing the likelihood of the participants responding to the researcher's agenda, making what they think is the preferred social response or behaving differently because of the presence of the researcher. However, the disadvantages of this strategy include the time and cost involved and the large volume of data produced, making prolonged engagement unfeasible for many researchers.

Central to a consideration of the length of time spent engaged in fieldwork is the issue of how the research developed over time, as this will be a determinant of study length. The dependability of interpretations may be threatened by premature closure of the analysis before data saturation has been achieved (Lincoln & Guba 1985).

Relating current findings to existing theories

The researcher may wish to demonstrate how the study findings support or contest existing theories and concepts (this is explored by Isabel Dyck in Chapter 8). Marshall and Rossman (1989) propose an explicit demonstration of how the research data tie into a body of theory, such that readers working within that theoretical framework may determine whether the case described could be transferred to other settings. However, Baxter and Eyles (1997) observe that appeals to conventional wisdom do not necessarily lead to rigorous findings, and may be counterproductive by serving to stifle more innovative thought and the development of 'new wisdom'.

Revisits to respondents to clarify meanings and verify interpretations

Central to the credibility of qualitative research is the ability of participants to recognize their own experiences and voice in the research findings (Krefting 1991), and so some researchers revisit respondents to clarify meanings and verify interpretations.

Krefting (1991) proposed that researchers should test their findings and interpretations against various groups or individuals from which the data were drawn, thus providing confidence that representations are faithful to the lived experiences perceived by the group. However, Hammersley (1992) is uneasy about efforts to ensure 'member-checking' of analytical constructs, observing that it is erroneous to assume that members of the study group have a 'privileged access to the truth' (p. 65). None the less, it must be emphasized that nor do researchers have a privileged access to the 'truth', and that 'whilst respondents do not have privileged access to the truth, they do have privileged access to their own opinions and meanings' (Baxter & Eyles 1997, p. 515). It is the adequate representation of these meanings that is the goal for member checking, and indeed for the qualitative research endeavour.

The strategy of involving all or some of the participants in a review of research materials ensures that the researcher has accurately translated their perspectives and decreases the chances of misrepresentation or appropriation. Member checking can be achieved in a variety of ways: participants may be given the opportunity to review and edit interview transcripts at an early stage, or they can be asked to react to a draft of the categories and themes derived as part of the data analysis process. Karen Hammell (Chapter 6) used this latter strategy to assist her in determining the authenticity of her analysis. She discussed at length theme definitions and the interpretations she was

making of the data with a participant who had expressed an interest in being involved.

Strategies that facilitate participant review assist in establishing the linkages between the researcher's constructs or interpretations and the original data. Noting that no single reality (or 'truth') exists, Baxter and Eyles (1997) suggest: 'It is not confirmation that is required from respondents as much as a commentary from them on the plausibility of the interpretations offered' (p. 512). Borlund (1991) suggests that without checking interpretations with the participants there is a danger of merely fitting data into existing theories with which we are comfortable. She suggests that there is also an ethical imperative to let study participants know how their narratives are going to be used.

Further, there may be conflicts between the researcher's conceptual framework, used to guide interpretations, and the participants' interpretations of their own lives. Although it is inevitable that people with different positions may have differing interpretations of reality, it is important to document these differences and discrepancies so that the reader can determine whether the researcher has imposed a viewpoint that is at odds with the participants' own understanding (see, for example, Borlund 1991). This relates to ethical issues of power and appropriation.

Attention to power relations involved in data collection process

Power within the research process has traditionally rested with the researchers – whether involved in quantitative or qualitative research – who usually control the design of the study, define the parameters of the theoretical framework and influence how the study is conducted, analysed and written up. It is from this position of power that researchers presume to represent the individuals or groups being researched.

Acker, Barry and Esseveld (1991) recognize that 'it is impossible to create a research process that erases the contradictions (in power and consciousness) between researcher and researched' (p. 150). Critics have provided an extensive discussion of the specifics of conducting ethical and responsible research (e.g. Olesen 1994). Central to these discussions is the concept of reciprocity, which implies give and take, a mutual negotiation of meaning and power in the research process. According to Lather (1991), this operates at two primary points in research: 'the junctures between researcher and researched and data and theory' (p. 57). Lather suggests that reciprocity could be facilitated by:

- conducting interviews in an interactive manner that requires self-disclosure on the part of the researcher
- conducting sequential interviews that allow a deeper probing of research issues
- negotiation between researcher and participant of the meanings embedded in the data by sharing interview transcripts, emerging themes and conclusions, and
- involving participants in identifying the research question and developing the research design.

These suggestions require a shift in our way of thinking about research design, but at the same time go a long way towards readdressing the power imbalances inherent in the researcher–participant relationship. Such strategies should be made transparent in the research report.

Ethical implications of representation and publication

How are data selected for presentation? Where are findings presented? How are participants' experiences represented? Is the researcher explicit about the purpose and agenda of the research? These are not just procedural issues, they are ethical issues.

The term 'representation' can be defined as a likeness, image, picture, description or account of an individual or group. Alcoff (1991) describes speaking and writing about others as 'the act of representing the other's needs, goals, situation, and in fact, *who they are*' (p. 9). The issue of representation raises questions of how accountability is established (and to whom we aim to be accountable), and demands the implementation of strategies designed to avoid the exploitation of research participants and the appropriation of their knowledge. These strategies must be outlined for the reader.

The concept of representation is interrelated with that of 'voice', about which important questions have been raised in qualitative research with respect to such data collection methods as interviews, oral histories and personal diaries. These questions focus on the meaning attributed by the researcher to what is said by the participant, the interpretation made as a result of what is said, and the space allowed within subsequent reports for the participants' voices to be heard. Again, the power of the researcher in making these choices should be made explicit.

In addition, any printed versions of the research are edited to fulfil a certain purpose and agenda, for example publication or conference presentation. The question becomes 'whose point of view is taken to report the findings' (Altheide & Johnson 1994, p. 486). The voice of the participant can be silenced through the editing process, and the role of the researcher in obtaining and analysing the data muted.

These and other ethical issues are clearly interrelated and are central to the qualitative research debate. It is the researcher's responsibility to ensure that the ethical implications of research are addressed in the design of the study and in disseminating the findings. The primary ethical considerations are those of adequately representing the participants' perspectives, and protecting their rights to privacy, confidentiality and protection from deceit and harm (see, for example, the process of ongoing consent obtained by Toby Wendland in Chapter 9, as the intended use for his subsequent report changed over time). Protection of human rights in qualitative research is achieved mainly by using the process of informed consent (which is the same method used in quantitative research). Informed consent is based on each participant being informed about all aspects of the research purpose and process, including risks and benefits, and clearly understanding that they can withdraw at any time. It can be argued that informed consent is inadequate for qualitative research because the direction the research will take is largely unknown at the beginning. However, as informed consent continues to be a requirement for ethical research practice, the authors of research articles need to make clear statements for the benefit of the critical reader about how the ethical issues were addressed in a particular study.

EVALUATION OF PUBLISHED RESEARCH

Discussion of strategies for the evaluation of qualitative research is particularly pertinent to the publishing of research findings in the form of articles. The points we have made relate to all forms of publications, although a thesis or book will have more space in which to provide a detailed account of all aspects of the research. In an article, space limitations will necessarily involve decisions on the writer's part concerning what should be included, and at what length. Authors may write several articles from one study, each emphasizing different aspects of the research. Given the space limitations of articles, and in order for the reader to have sufficient detail by which a reasoned evaluation of the research may be made, the article must be well organized and clearly written (see, for example, McCuaig & Frank 1991).

There are many ways to write up research findings. The specific components of a report may vary, but they all need:

Box 10.2 Framework of evaluative guidelines for evaluating published research

When critically reading an article, consider:
- Appropriateness of methodology and consistency of interpretation
- Strategies for enhancing the rigour of the research employed:
  - The researcher role: positionality and reflexivity
  - Triangulation
  - Period of time spent with participants
  - Participant review of findings and interpretations
  - Peer review
  - Ethical implications of the research.

Introductory material
- Is the purpose of the article and/or the objective of the study clearly stated?
- Is a background to the study provided? (which provides some context of the problem and makes the importance of the study clear)
- Is the researcher's particular interest in the study clearly identified?
- Is a statement made of what the article will argue?

Body of the article
- Is there a review of related literature?
- Are the researcher's theoretical perspective or conceptual framework and/or assumptions identified?
- Is the research methodology appropriate for the purposes of the study?
- Is an account of the research process given? This could include type and setting of study,

length of study, participant recruitment criteria or method of selection stated, selection of methods and nature of data, researcher–participant relations, progress of research. In other words, can the reader follow the decision-trail of the researcher in concept development and/or presentation of argument?
- What sort of evidence is provided for generalized findings, e.g. does the researcher make a general statement and illustrate it with primary participant quotes?

Discussion and conclusion
- Does the discussion relate back to the initial problem/question and relevant literature?
- Are any practical and/or theoretical implications of the research considered?
- Are any limitations of the research identified?
- Are any recommendations for future research made?

References
- Are these complete and up to date both in the text and in the reference list?

In summary
- Do you know why this research was carried out?
- Was it systematic?
- Does the article help you to understand the phenomenon in question better?
- Is the article clearly written and logically organized?

- an introduction, which provides information on the subject matter of the article and what it will include
- the body of the article, which presents, explains and argues the researcher's main points, and
- a concluding section that summarizes the main points, draws the arguments together and suggests implications for practice and/or further research.

Box 10.2 illustrates a framework of evaluative guidelines (adapted from material developed by Isabel Dyck for an undergraduate course: 'Introduction to Scientific Inquiry: Qualitative Methodology') providing suggestions for critical reading of qualitative research papers.

CONCLUSION

It is important to reiterate that, although there can be no mandatory rules for gauging the merits of qualitative research, there clearly need to be 'criteria that enable a judgement to be made concerning honesty, integrity and plausibility of design and accounts' (Baxter & Eyles 1997, p. 521). We submit that the criteria outlined in this chapter should be understood to be general, and thus may be satisfied in different ways, congruent with the nature and purpose of each study. Our goal must be to achieve a high standard of qualitative research which will contribute to the knowledge bases of our professions, and thereafter enhance the service we provide to our clients.

REFERENCES

Acker J, Barry K, Esseveld J 1991 Objectivity and truth: problems in doing feminist research. In: Fonow M, Cook J (eds) Beyond methodology: feminist scholarship as lived research. Indiana University Press, Bloomington, pp 133–153
Agar M 1986 Speaking of ethnography. Sage, Beverley Hills
Alcoff L 1991 The problem of speaking for others. Cultural Critique Winter: 5–31
Altheide DL, Johnson JM 1994 Criteria for assessing interpretive validity in qualitative research. In: Denzin N,

Lincoln Y (eds) Handbook of qualitative research. Sage, Thousand Oaks, pp 485–498
Atkinson P 1990 The ethnographic imagination: textual constructions of reality. Routledge, London
Baxter J, Eyles J 1997 Evaluating qualitative research in social geography: establishing 'rigour' in interview analysis. Transactions of the Institute of British Geographers 22(4):505–525
Bogdan RC, Biklen SK 1998 Qualitative research for education: an introduction to the theory and methods, 3rd edn. Allyn & Bacon, Boston
Borlund K 1991 'That's not what I said': Interpretive conflict in oral narrative research. In: Gluck SB, Patai D (eds) Women's words. The feminist practice of oral history. Routledge, New York, pp 63–76
Clifford C 1997 Qualitative research methodology in nursing and healthcare. Churchill Livingstone, Edinburgh
Domholdt E 1993 Research paradigms. In: Domholdt E. Physical therapy research: principles and applications. WB Saunders, Philadelphia, pp 121–140
Gliner JA 1994 Reviewing qualitative research: proposed criteria for fairness and rigor. Occupational Therapy Journal of Research 14(2):78–90
Guba EG 1981 Criteria for assessing the trustworthiness of naturalistic inquiries. Education Communication and Technology Journal 29:75–91
Hammersley M 1992 What's wrong with ethnography? Routledge, London
Hasselkus BR 1991 Qualitative research: not another orthodoxy. Occupational Therapy Journal of Research 11(1):3–7
Krefting L 1991 Rigor in qualitative research: the assessment of trustworthiness. American Journal of Occupational Therapy 45(3):214–222
Lather P 1991 Getting smarter: feminist research and pedagogy with/in the postmodern. Routledge, New York
Lincoln YS, Guba EG 1985 Naturalistic inquiry. Sage, Beverley Hills
McCuaig M, Frank G 1991 The able self: adaptive patterns and choices in independent living for a person with cerebral palsy. American Journal of Occupational Therapy 45(3):224–234
Marshall C, Rossman GB 1989 Designing qualitative research. Sage, Newbury Park
Mays N Pope C 1995 Rigour and qualitative research. British Medical Journal 311:109–112
Morse JM, Field PA 1995 Qualitative research methods for health professionals. Sage, Thousand Oaks
Oakley A 1981 Interviewing women: a contradiction in terms. In: Roberts H (ed) Doing feminist research. Routledge, London, pp 30–61
Olesen V 1994 Feminisms and models of qualitative research. In: Denzin N K, Lincoln YS (eds) Handbook of qualitative research. Sage, London, pp 158–174
Punch M (1994) Politics and ethics in qualitative research. In: Denzin N K, Lincoln YS (eds) Handbook of qualitative research. Sage, London, pp 83–97
Robson C 1993 Real world research. A resource for social scientists and practitioner-researchers. Blackwell, Oxford

Sandelowski M 1986 The problem of rigor in qualitative research. Advances in Nursing Science 8:27–37

Strauss AL, Corbin J 1990 Basics of qualitative research. Sage, Newbury Park

FURTHER READING

Barnes C, Mercer G (eds) 1997 Doing disability research. Disability Press, Leeds

Bhavnani K-K 1993 Tracing the contours. Feminist research and feminist objectivity. Women's Studies International Forum 16(2):95–104

England K 1994 Getting personal: reflexivity, positionality and feminist research. Professional Geographer 46(1):80–89

Fine M 1994 Working the hyphens: reinventing self and other in qualitative research. In: Denzin NK, Lincoln YS (eds) Handbook of qualitative research. Sage, London, pp 70–82

Index